STRENGTH TRAINING

FOR LIFE

A Complete Guide to Increase Your Energy and Reverse the Aging Process After 40 + Building Muscle for Beginners: The Complete Blueprint to Building Muscle with Weight Lifting

3 Books In 1

Baz Thompson

Table of Content

Book 1

Strength Training After 40:

101 Exercises for Seniors to Maximize Energy
and Improve Flexibility and Mobility with

90-Day Workout Plan

INTRODUCTION

Do you think it is too late to build muscle and Strength after 45? Well, if your answer is a "Yes," then you might want to rethink your response in a bit!

The actual truth is that age-related changes like slower metabolism rate, shrinking of your muscle mass, and the decline of hormonal and neurological responses are bound to begin at middle age. That's precisely how our bodies are built. However, when you begin to focus on improving your fitness performance, primarily through strength training, then, believe me, magic will happen!

Working consistently and diligently towards building and maintaining your body strength comes with many beneficial packages. It helps you keep your bones healthy, thereby reducing pain from arthritis which most seniors tend to deal with as they grow older. You can also easily improve your body's mobility and stability while working your legs to prevent occasional falls and hip fractures common with older people. Being regularly active also transforms to a lowered risk of several chronic conditions and illnesses. Now you can see that exercising can be a fun and rewarding way to stay active even as a senior. Fortunately, you don't have to spend hundreds of dollars on a lengthy course to get all these benefits. This book has compiled 101 highly-effective strength training exercises that can help you reach the highest point of your fitness performance.

This book is also designed to be your ultimate guide as you begin your quest to build muscle and Strength in almost the same way younger people do. At this point, I wish you a lovely time as you read and internalize the contents of this book!

101 Workouts to Improve Balance and Stability, Restore Strength, and Enjoy an Active Lifestyle.

Before getting started with any of the exercises that we will soon be discussing, let's talk about some tips that will surely help you as seniors.

Firstly, if you can afford it, you might want to get professional advice. Though most of these exercises can be performed with or without a therapist but in the most severe cases, your physical therapist must be comfortable and confident that you're able to safely do the exercises.

Staying hydrated is another necessity! Most older people tend to drink less water to avoid multiple trips to the bathroom. However, to achieve maximum results without putting yourself in danger, you must drink water before and after exercising.

In the same way, you must understand that it is impossible to out-exercise a low diet. Eating a well-balanced meal before and after a workout will undoubtedly lead to a better outcome!

Nevertheless, for every one of these exercises, having a proper form should be your primary focus. It is only by doing so that you will reap the benefits of whatever types of strength training exercise you do.

Keep in mind that patience, determination, and consistency are vital things you must-have for this journey! Now that we have sorted the basic tips out let's get started!

PART ONE: BUILDING

MUSCLES

Arms

Biceps Curl

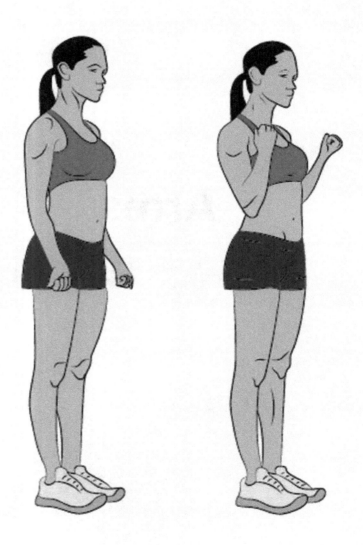

1. Biceps Curl

Biceps curls are standard foundational exercises for building the muscles of the arm. By strengthening these muscles, you are also improving the stability of the motion of your arms and hands, especially when carrying anything of significance.

- Other Targeted Areas: Forearms and some of your shoulder muscles, including your deltoids.
- Length of workout: 10 minutes x Time duration for resting periods: 30 to 90 seconds between each set.
- Estimated calorie burns: Doing about three sets of 12 bicep curl repetitions, especially with dumbbells, you are most likely to burn up to 25 calories.

Instructions

- Get a sturdy chair and sit up tall with your hands positioned at your sides and your palms forward.
- Now focus on your arm while keeping your shoulder in; back straight, and your core tight. Focus on your biceps.
- Maintain this position and curl your arm from the elbow, all the way up to the top, and then slowly lower it back down.
- Ensure that you keep your shoulder from rotating as you completely straighten your arm on the way down and fully bend it on the way up.
- Breathing: Inhale while lifting your arm and exhale during the downward movement phase.

Level up: To make this exercise more challenging, you can hold dumbbells in your two hands and follow these instructions. For a beginner, it is recommended that you start with a two pounds dumbbell.

Precautions

- Be gentle and don't rush as it is not how fast you are that matters. What's important is your ability to perform the movement correctly.
- Go as high as comfortable.

Lateral Raise

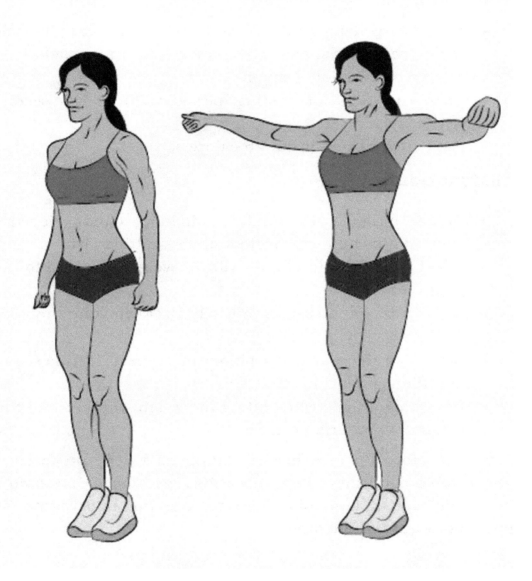

2. Lateral Raise

Upright rows are a set of upper body exercises that increase the Strength in your upper arms, thereby improving your ability to lift heavier loads.

- Other targeted areas: All your three shoulder muscles (delts, rhomboids, and teres minor) and upper back.
- Length of workout: 7 mins
- Time duration for resting periods: 30 to 40 seconds between each set.
- Estimated calorie burn: 25 calories.

Instructions

- Stand upright with dumbbells-holding hands placed in front of hips and your feet shoulder-width apart.
- While bending your elbows, lift the weights upward toward your chin.
- Make sure you do not arch the back. Keep your shoulders down.
- Return to the starting position and repeat 10 times. Rest and then go for 2 more sets.
- Breathing: inhale while lifting the weight upward and then exhale as you bring it down.

Level up: Move up to a heavier dumbbell when you feel very comfortable performing more than 20 repetitions. Or switch to an elastic band and try doing these same motion upper arms with one foot in front of the other.

Precautions

- Keep your spine straight through the movement.
- Make sure the dumbbells are not too heavy or disturbing your form

Tricep Extension

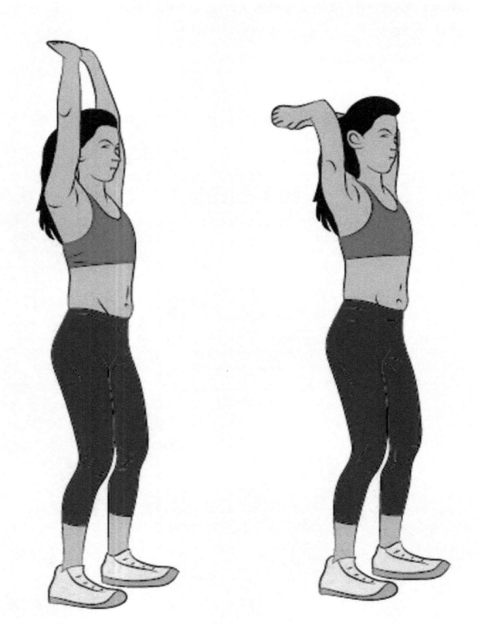

3. Triceps Extension

As you've obviously detected from the name, this exercise aims to strengthen your triceps – the muscles in the back of the upper arms. The triceps muscles are involved in pretty much everything you do with your hand.

- Length of workout: 6 mins
- Time duration for resting periods: 20 to 30 seconds between sets.
- Estimated calorie burn: 16 calories

Instruction

- Sit tall in a sturdy chair with your back straight, feet flat on the floor, and legs about hip-width apart.
- Hold one hand in a tight fist, then bring your arm straight up, reaching towards the ceiling.
- Place your other hand just below the elbow of the extended arm for support.
- Now slowly lower your extended arm down and hide it behind your head.
- Bring the arm back up to the starting position. That's one rep!
- Now go ahead and do about 8-12 reps and then switch arms. To achieve effective results, aim for 3 sets of the 8-12 reps.

Level up: While these instructions are just based on your body weight, you can also go through the same motion with an extra resistance by using 1–3-pound dumbbell weights depending on your strength level.

Precautions

- Only reach your hand as high as comfortable. Pause and lower it a little bit if you begin to Precautions
- Make sure to inhale during the upward movement and exhale while lowering your hand down.

Lat Pull with Band

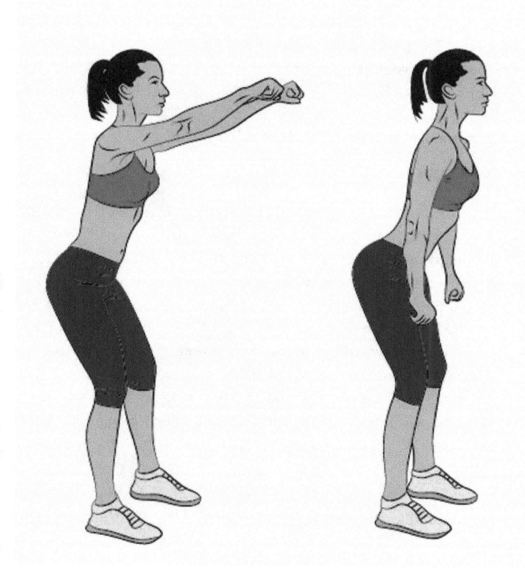

4. Lat Pull with Band

Though this exercise primarily works your lats muscles on either side of the back, it also strengthens your biceps and forearms. They also provide crucial support and stability to your spine.

- Other Targeted Areas: side shoulders, back.
- Length of workout: 9 minutes
- Time duration for resting periods: 30secs -1 minutes in-between each set
- Estimated calorie burn: 36 calories.

Instructions

- Sit up and place the resistance band around your wrists.
- Raise your hands over your head in a shoulder-width position so that there is tension on the band.
- Make sure your back is flat, and your abs are engaged.
- While keeping your left hand in place, squeeze the muscles on the right side of your back to pull the elbow of your right hand down towards your rib cage. Keep it slow. x Pause for 2 seconds and then press it back up.
- Go for 5 reps on the right side, then switch sides and do 5 reps on the left side. Go for another set of 5 reps on each side.

Precautions

Keep your back as straight as possible throughout the movement.

Wall Push-Ups

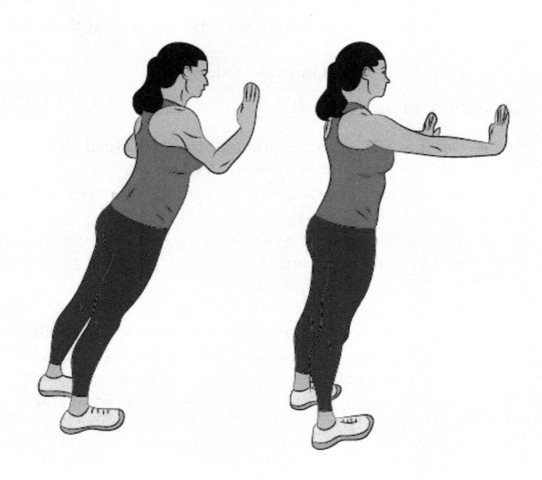

5. Wall Push-Ups

With this set of push-ups, you don't have to worry about struggling to get down on the floor and then being stuck there! Wall push-ups target and strengthen your entire upper body with a great amount of focus on your arms.

- Other target areas: Chest, back, and shoulders.
- Length of workout: 10 mins
- Time duration for resting periods: 1 to 2 minutes between sets
- Estimated calorie burn: 40 calories.

Instructions

- Get into a standing position in front of a sturdy wall, up to two feet away but as close as you need to.
- Stretch your hands directly in front of your shoulders and place them against the wall.
- Ensure that your body is in straight form. Engage your core and breathe in as you bend your elbows slowly to lean in with your chest towards the wall.
- Pause when your face is close to the wall and then exhale slowly as you straighten your arms to push your body away from the wall. That's a complete one rep
- Always remember to concentrate on this form as you go further. Keep your back and ensure that your hips don't sag.
- Go for 3 sets of 10 reps while taking rest in-between the sets.

Level up: To make the exercise more challenging, you don't really need any equipment. Just take one more step away from the wall;

keep your feet shoulder-width apart, and then repeat the same motions.

Precautions

- Don't bend your elbows too much as you lean in towards the wall.
- Keep breathing properly.

Wall Angels

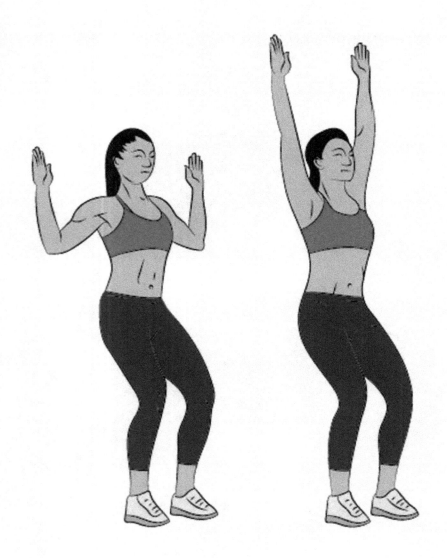

6. Wall Angels

Constantly looking downwards increases tightness in your chest and middle area. What this exercise does to remedy that is to open up your chest and relieve the tension in your upper back.

- Other targeted areas: Arms, neck
- Length of workout: 6 mins
- Time duration for resting periods: 30 – 40 secs in-between each set.
- Estimated calorie burn: 25 calories

Instructions

- Stand in front of a wall with your head, lower back, and butt flat against it.
- Place your hands at your sides with the back of your palms out and against the wall.
- While keeping your arms in touch with the wall, raise them as high as is comfortable, preferably above your head.
- Slowly, bring it back down. As you go up and down, keep imagining that you're making some beautiful imaginary wings for your angel.
- Perform 3 sets of 10 repetitions.
- Try as much as possible not to lift your hips or protrude your neck during this exercise. Keep it slow!

Level up: Up for a challenge? Practice doing a hollow-sit together with the Wall Angel movement.

Precautions

- Don't place your hands too high up the wall

Hands

The following hand exercises will help target and strengthen your arms, wrists, fingers, and palm. But before actually performing any of these exercises, we have a good idea for warming up your hands that you don't want to miss!

It is pretty simple. Just use a microwave hot pack on your hands and palm. This will increase the temperature of the tissues, ligaments, and tendons, under your skin, making them much more elastic. Try it and see how much further and easier you can open and close your hand.

Finger Bends

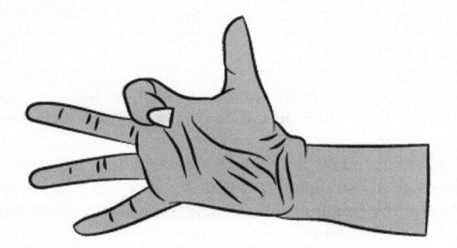

7. Finger Bends

Finger Bends are a simple home exercise that keeps the joints in your fingers moving against the deterioration in hand function that is common with old age.

- Other targeted areas: Arms
- Length of workout: 8 minutes
- The time duration for resting periods: 10 secs break in-between sets
- Estimated calorie burn: 21 calories.

Instructions

- Start by holding your right hand up and straight.
- Slowly, bend your thumb down towards the direction of your palm.
- Hold the bend for two to six seconds.
- Then gently straighten out your thumb.
- Repeat the bending and releasing movement on each finger on your right hand.
- Repeat the entire sequence on the opposite hand.
- Repeat the entire movement for 4 times on both hands. Take a break and then perform another set of 4 repetitions on both hands.

Precautions

- Don't bend too hard and release the hold once you begin to feel pain

Make a Fist

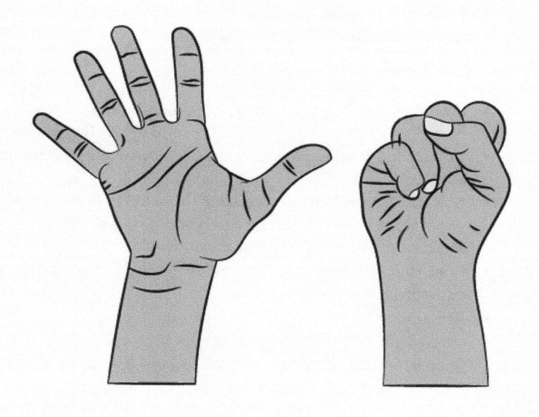

8. Make a Fist

The "Make A Fist" movement can help strengthen the muscles of your hands and fingers while increasing your range of motion and giving you pain relief simultaneously.

- Other targeted areas: wrist, and forearms
- Length of workout: 6 mins
- Time duration for resting periods: 10 secs in-between sets
- Estimated calorie burn: 19 calories.

Instructions

- Start by holding your right hand up and straight. Think of it as if you were going to give someone a "Hi-five" shake.
- Ensure that you keep your wrist and forearm close to a flat surface.
- Now, close your fingers together to make a gentle fist with your thumb wrapped across your fingers. Try not to squeeze your fingers into your palms.
- Hold that position for 10 to 30 seconds. x Slowly release and spread your fingers wide.
- Remember to stretch only until you feel tightness. You should not be feeling pain so pause if it seems so.
- Repeat at least 5 times on both hands and then go for 3 more sets.

Precautions

- Release the clenched fingers when you begin to feel pain.
- Try not to squeeze your fingers too much into your palm.

Thumb Bends

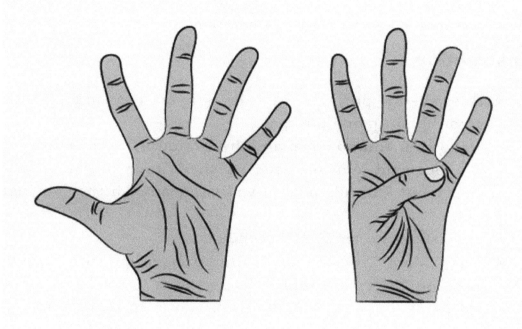

9. Thumb Bends

This exercise is just like the finger bends, except that here, we will be concentrating only on your thumbs.

- Other targeted areas: Wrist and Forearms
- Length of workout: 6 mins
- Time duration for resting periods: 10-20 secs in-between each set.
- Estimated calorie burn: 21 calories

Instructions

- Just like the previous two exercises, start by holding your right hand up and straight.
- Bend your thumb down and inward toward your palm.
- As you bend, aim to reach for the bottom of your pinky finger but still, it's okay if you cannot reach that far just yet.
- Hold the bend for 5 -10 seconds.
- Then slowly release your thumb back to the starting position. That's one rep!
- Repeat 5 times on both your left and right hand. Then go for 3 more sets!

Precautions

- Don't bend your thumbs too much to the point of pain.

Make a "C"

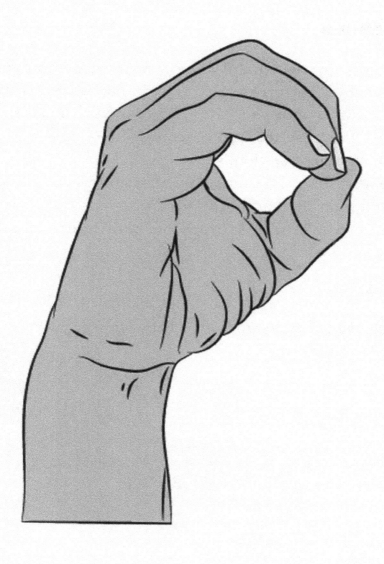

10. Make a "C"

- Length of workout: 5 mins
- Time duration for resting periods: 5 secs in-between sets
- Estimated calorie burn: 19 calories.

Instructions

- Start your right hand extended upwards and your fingers straight. To create a "C" shape, curve your fingers downward with your thumb out and to the side.
- Hold the pose for 2 to 5 seconds x Release and Return to the starting position.
- Repeat about 10 times on your right hand
- Switch on the left hand and do 10 reps.
- Perform 3 sets of 10 reps on both hands; resting where necessary.

Precautions

- Release the hold when you begin to feel pain

Finger Lifts

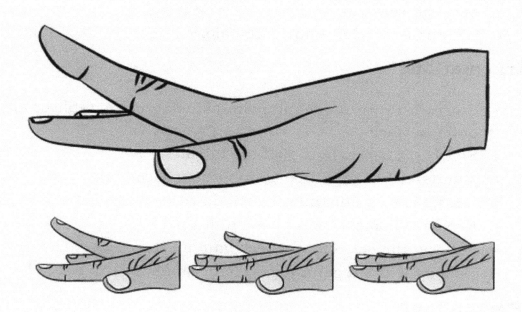

11. Finger Lifts

This simple exercise helps to strengthen your hands and fingers. It also improves your flexibility and mobility level by expanding your range of motion.

- x Length of workout: 8 min
- x Time duration for resting periods: 10 to 20 secs in-between sets.
- x Estimated calorie burn: 16 calories.

Instructions

- Start with your hand and palm-side flat on the table or any other surface.
- Slowly, lift your thumb off the table.
- Maintain that raised position for two seconds.
- Gently lower your thumb back down.
- Repeat this movement on each finger.
- Perform the entire sequence again on the opposite hand.
- Do 2 sets of 5 repetitions on both hands.

Precautions

- Only lift each finger as high as you're comfortable.

Wrist Stretches

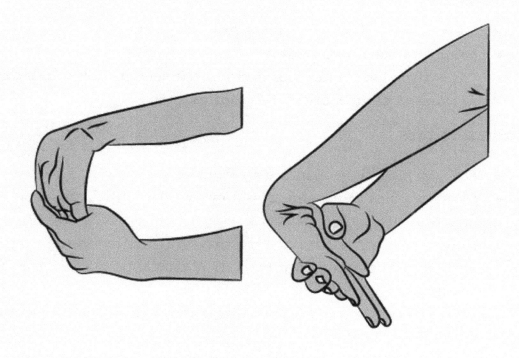

12. Wrist Stretches

Wrist pain, weakness, and stiffness are common problems for seniors. However, practicing simple wrist stretches movement is an easy and effective way to strengthen your wrists and keep your hands and fingers flexible. It also helps to lower the risk of injuries in your wrist area.

- Other targeted areas: fingers and forearms.
- Length of workout: 4 mins
- Time duration for resting periods: 10 secs in-between sets
- Estimated calorie burn: 15 calories.

Instructions

- Extend your right arm out in front of you
- Slowly, point your fingers downwards until you feel a stretch.
- Now, use your left hand to gently pull the extended hand and finger toward your body. Hold this position for 3–5 seconds.
- Release and then point your fingers toward the ceiling until you feel a stretch.
- Use the left hand again to gently pull the raised hand toward the body. Hold this position for 3–5 seconds.
- Repeat this five times and then alternate arms
- Do 2 more sets of 5 reps on both arms.

Precautions

- Stop when you feel pain.

Give the Okay

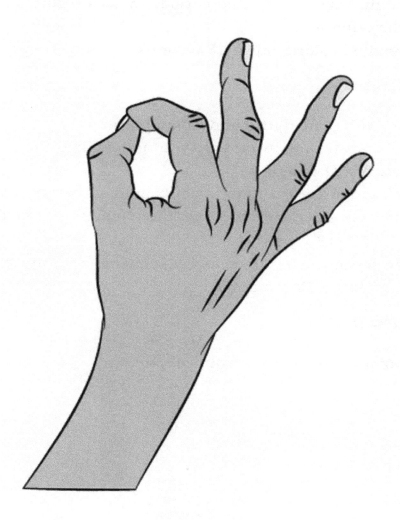

13. Give the Okay

The "Give the Okay" exercise is very effective when it comes to reducing arthritis pains in your fingers. It also stretches and strengthens your finger muscles.

- Length of workout: 4 mins
- Time duration for resting periods: 5 secs before switching to the other arm.
- Estimated calorie burn: 15 calories.

Instructions

- Start with your right hand up and straight.
- Turn your thumb inwards to your index fingertip. It should create an "O" shape
- Next, touch your thumb to your middle fingertip and then repeat the same movement on the remaining three fingers.
- Go for 10 -12 reps.
- Then repeat the entire exercise sequence on your left hand for the same 10 -12 times.

Precautions

- Relax and pause when you feel pain.

Ball Squeezes

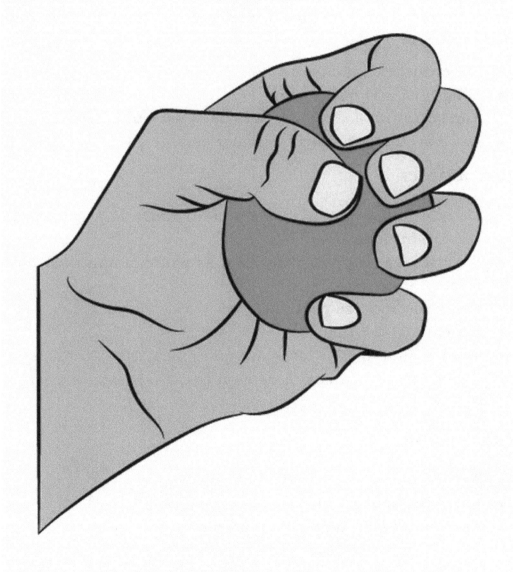

14. Ball Squeezes

Ball squeezes are simple wrist strengthening exercises that you can do while watching TV or relaxing in the garden. Asides from strengthening your grips, these stretches also help combat carpal tunnel, arthritis, and pain or weakness in your wrist and finger areas.

- Other targeted areas: Arms
- Length of workout: 3 mins
- Time duration for resting periods: 5 secs in between sets
- Estimated calorie burn: 21 calories.

Instructions

- Hold a tennis ball or just a small rubber or foam ball in your right hand.
- Slowly squeeze the ball as hard as you can and then hold it for 3-5 seconds.
- Relax the squeeze gently.
- Repeat 10 – 15 times.
- Then switch to your left hand and repeat 10 – 15 times
- Repeat 10 – 15 times more with the two hands; making it 2 sets.

Precautions

- Avoid using a very hardball at all cost
- Relax the squeeze slowly
- Assisted Finger abductions stretch

Assisted Finger Abductions Stretch

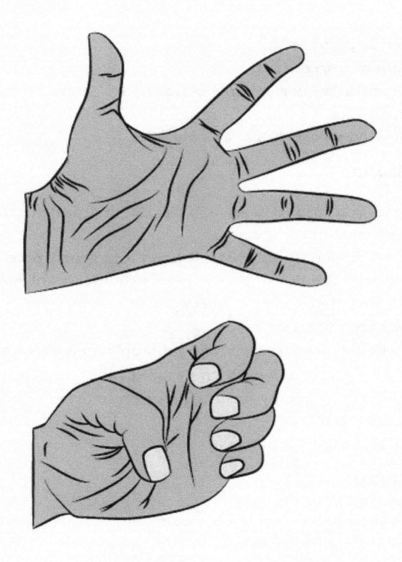

15. Assisted Finger Abductions Stretch

This exercise targets the muscles between each of your fingers which are often ignored. By stretching and strengthening them, the mobility and flexibility of the fingers eventually improve.

- Other targeted areas: Forearms.
- Length of workout: 10 mins
- Time duration for resting periods: 5-10 secs in-between sets.
- Estimated calorie burn: 15 calories.

Instructions

- Extend your right hand a little bit in front of you and spread your five fingers
- Use two fingers from your left hand and gently press them in between the two fingers of your extended right hand.
- Make sure that the two fingers you are using from your left hands are in scissor mode.
- You should feel the stretch as you apply a bit of resistance.
- Hold for 5 seconds and then switch to the next finger.
- Do the same for all your fingers before moving to your left hands.
- Do 3 sets of 5 repetitions.

Precautions

- If you can keep your hand steady enough, use a table for support.

Hand Open/Closes

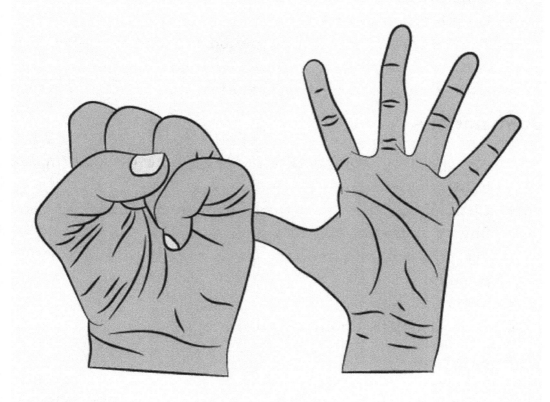

16. Hand Open/Closes

This simple exercise of clenching your fist and spreading your fingers helps to increase the Strength of your finger. It also helps to loosen up tight fingers and lowers the risk of injury.

- Other targeted areas: Forearms
- Length of workout: 4 mins
- Time duration for resting periods: 5-10secs in-between sets.
- Estimated calorie burn: 15 calories.

Instructions

- Sit with your arms extending upwards with your fingers beside your head.
- Clench your fist tight, then open up by spreading your fingers as far as you can.
- Try to make your movements as controlled and slow as possible.
- Repeat 10 times.
- Then complete 4 more sets of 10 reps.

Precautions

- Open up your hands as far as comfortable. Stop when it gets painful

Thumb Flexions

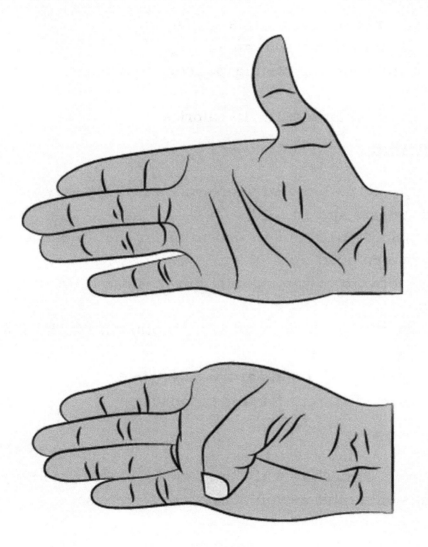

17. Thumb Flexions

This exercise basically targets your thumbs. The idea here is that by working your thumb, the Strength, mobility, and flexibility in those muscles will increase.

- Other targeted areas: Arms
- Length of workout: 4 minutes
- Time duration for resting periods: 5-10 secs in-between sets.
- Estimated calorie burn: 19 calories.

Instructions

- Sit upright and extend your arms a little bit forward with your fingers spread.
- Now, slowly use your thumb to touch the tip of the index finger then open up.
- Move forward to your middle finger, close it up with your thumb and then open up.
- Repeat till you have used your thumb to touch all your other four fingers.
- You can do both hands at the same time.
- Do 2 sets of 10 reps for this exercise.

Precautions

- If you're struggling with hand joints problems, rest your hands on a table as you perform this exercise.

Wrist Flexion

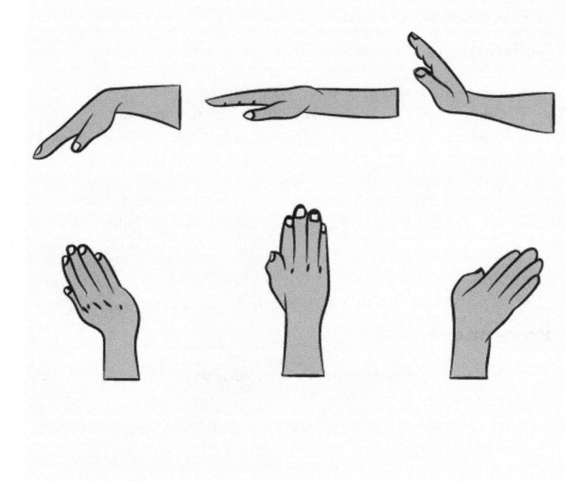

18. Wrist Flexion

Wrist flexion is not just a strengthening-training exercise. It also serves as a wrist tension and pain reliever for seniors!

- Other targeted areas: Arms
- Length of workout: 5 mins
- Time duration for resting periods: 10-20 secs in between sets.
- Estimated calorie burn: 15 calories.

Instructions

- Get seated and stretch forth your right arm
- Clench your fist but make sure it is not too tight.
- Now move your wrist up and down. Keep doing that for 10 seconds.
- When you feel it too uncomfortable, you can use your other arm to support it.
- Release your fingers and then repeat the movement 5 more times.
- Switch to your other arm and do the same.
- Do 3 sets of 5 reps on each wrist.

Precautions

- Use your other arm to support your wrist as you go up and down.
- Pause and stop if you begin to feel pain.

Wrist Radial

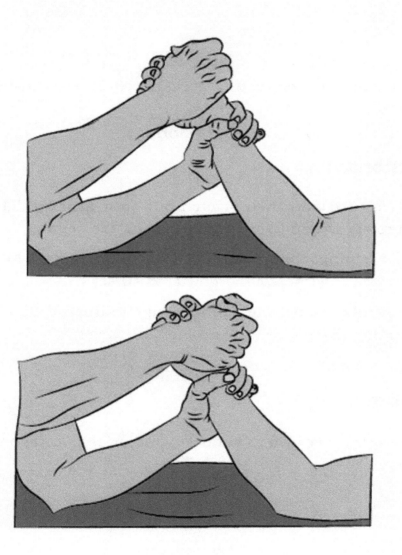

19. Wrist Radial

This exercise basically offers the same as the wrist flexion exercise. You would also see the similarities in both exercise routines.

- Other targeted areas: Arms
- Length of workout: 5 mins
- Time duration for resting periods: 10-20 secs in-between sets.
- Estimated calorie burn: 15 calories.

Instructions

Get seated and then stretch out your arm straight with your fingers spread and your thumb facing the ceiling.

Maintaining that position, clench your fist and then slowly move your wrist up and down for 10 secs.

Remember to use your other arm for support. You should feel the stretch from your forearms to your wrist.

Do 3 sets of 5 reps on each wrist.

Precautions

- Use your other arm to support your wrist as you go up and down.

Elbow Flexion

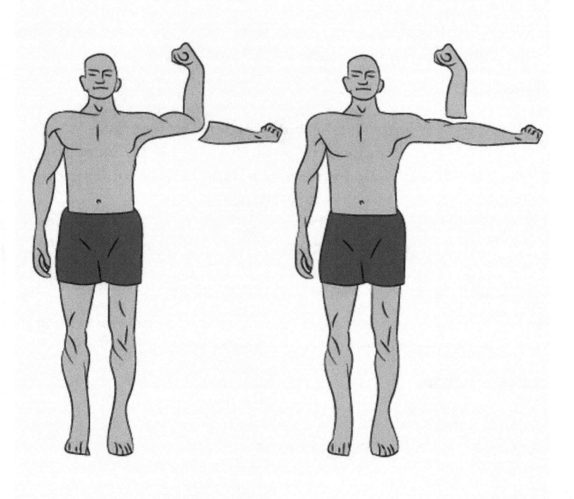

20. Elbow Flexion

Elbow flexion simply means your ability to bend your elbow. This exercise helps to expand your elbow range of motion, which in turn improves your ability to fully bend your elbows.

- Other targeted areas: Wrist and forearm.
- Length of workout: 5 mins
- Time duration for resting periods: 20 secs in-between sets
- Estimated calorie burn: 19 calories.

Instructions

- Stand up and straight with your arm at your side.
- Actively but gently bend your elbow up as far as possible.
- Then, grasp your forearm or wrist with your other straight hand and gently add resistance.
- Hold the bent position of your elbow for 5 to 10 seconds.
- Release the stretch by straightening your elbow.
- Repeat the exercise 5 times. Take a rest and then go for 2 more sets of the same 5 reps movement.

Level up: You can add a bit of stretch to your elbow flexion exercise by holding onto a 2- to 3-pound weight.

Precautions

- Be gentle as you bend your elbows
- Only go as far as you feel comfortable

Elbow Pronation

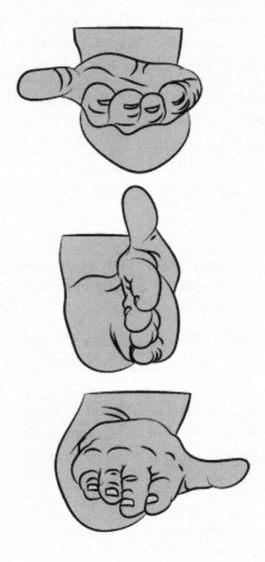

21. Elbow Pronation

Aging is associated with elbow pain which can often limit your ability to perform basic functional tasks. Being consistent with the elbow pronation exercise helps improve your ability to turn your hand over so your palm faces the floor. This motion makes it absolutely convenient for you to do tasks like pouring a cup of coffee or playing the piano.

- Other targeted areas: Wrists and forearm
- Length of workout: 5 mins
- Time duration for resting periods: 20 to 30 secs between each set.
- Estimated calorie burn: 19 calories.

Instructions

Sit up in a sturdy chair with your elbow bent 90 degrees and tucked in at your side. x Slowly, turn your hand and wrist over as far as possible,

- Then reach your other hand over the top of your forearm to grab your wrist, and turn your arm further into a pronated position.
- Hold the position with a little bit of resistance for five to 10 seconds. Repeat the exercise 5 times. Take a rest and then go for 2 more sets of the same 5 reps movement.

Precautions

- Only maintain the pronated position for as long as you feel comfortable.

Shoulder Strengthening

Training

Shrug

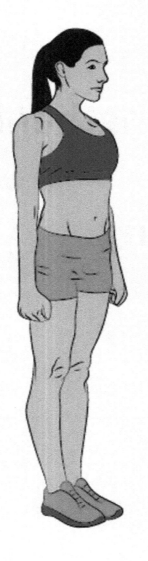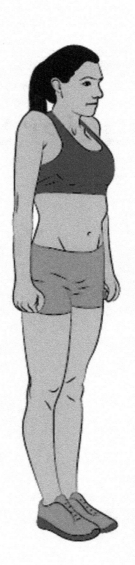

22. Shoulder Shrug

This exercise targets your scapula which is the triangle bone in the back of your shoulder. It also helps to improve the Strength, mobility, and stability of your shoulder blades. Interestingly, having a strong scapula basically translates to having functional and strong arms suitable for heavier lifting. So, let's give it a try!

- Other targeted areas: Neck and upper back muscles.
- Length of workout: 10 mins
- Time duration for resting periods: 20 to 30 secs x Estimated calorie burn: 31 calories.

Instructions

- Get dumbbells that you are very comfortable with but try not to overdo them.
- Sit up with the dumbbells in your hands, your arms by your sides, and feet shoulder width apart.
- Now try to keep your elbows fully extended as you raise your shoulders upward slowly toward your ears. Go as high as you can, then pause for a 2-sec count. x Exhale as you move your shoulder backward and down to return to the starting position.
- To make this motion easier, ensure that you lift your ribcage and slightly flex your knees. Also, tuck in your chin.
- Repeat 4 sets of 5 repetitions.

Level up: To take it a step more intense, try this shoulder shrug exercise while standing to increase your balance. Also, take up a heavier weight when you can perform more than 20 repetitions with no stress. Or you can switch to an elastic band.

Precautions

- Don't raise your shoulder beyond the point you feel is safe.

Kneeling Shoulder Tap Push Up

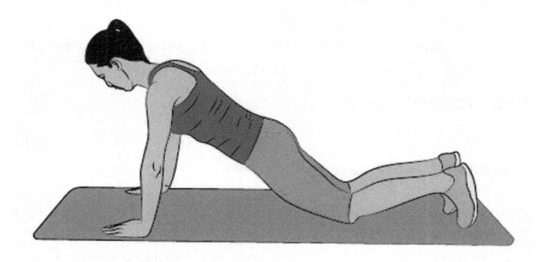

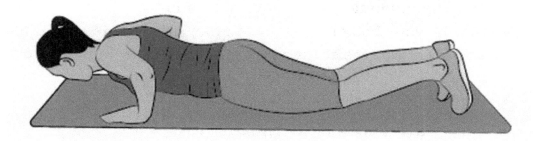

23. Kneeling Shoulder Tap Push Up

This is an excellent bodyweight exercise for building muscle and Strength in the upper body. Along with targeting your shoulders, it also improves your entire body balance and stability level.

- Other targeted areas: arms, chest, back, shoulders, core
- Length of workout: 5 minutes
- Time duration for resting periods: 20 secs in-between sets.
- Estimated calorie burn: 25 calories.

Instructions

- Get into a kneeling plank position with your hands on the ground beneath your shoulders and your back extended long to the knees.
- Slowly lower your chest to the floor, keeping your core very tight.
- As you push back up to the kneeling plank position, tap your left shoulder with your right hand, then set it down.
- Repeat the push-up motion but this time, as you rise tap your right shoulder with your left hand.
- Surely, your body may want to sway side to side as you lift and lower but resist the urge to do so by keeping your core tight.
- Perform 3 sets of 4 reps each.

Level up: Switch to heavier weights.

Precautions

- Keep your core tight so that your form remains strict.
- Breathe properly in through your nose and out through your mouth.

Finger Marching

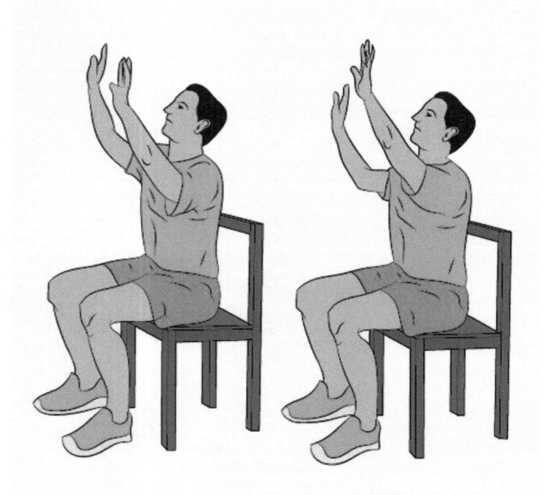

24. Finger Marching

Legs are basically for movement, but in this exercise, your fingers, hands, and arms will do the walking. The Finger Marching movement is designed to strengthen your upper body as well as improve the flexibility of your shoulders and other muscle groups close to that area.

- Other targeted areas: Arms and back
- Length of workout: 4 mins
- Time duration for resting periods: 5-10 secs in-between sets.
- Estimated calorie burn: 21 calories.

Instructions

- Get a sturdy armless chair and sit forward with your feet on the floor, shoulder-width apart.
- Now, imagine there is a wall directly in front of you. Slowly walk your fingers up the wall until your arms are extended above your head.
- Hold your wiggling fingers in that overhead position for about ten seconds and then slowly walk them back down.
- To know if you're doing this, you should be feeling a stretch in your back, arms, and chest.
- Repeat this exercise 10 times, rest, and then go for another set of 10 repetitions.

Precaution

- If you're unable to march your finger till overhead, just stop where it is comfortable and march them back down.

Shoulder Overhead Press

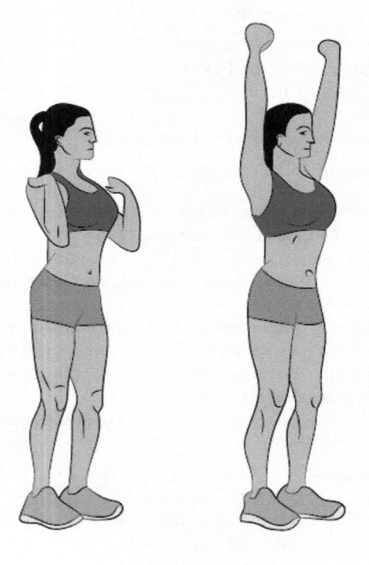

25. Shoulder Overhead Press

If you're still determined about adding size and Strength to your shoulders even as a senior, then this is another must-do shoulder-strengthening exercise that basically works your upper body to help you achieve that dream! x Other targeted areas: biceps, back.

- Length of workout: 5 mins
- Time duration for resting periods: Rest for 20 secs in between sets
- Estimated calorie burn: 20 calories.

Instructions

- Start with dumbbells in your hands and your feet hip-distance apart.
- Now stretch your elbows out to the side creating a goal post position with arms.
- Your dumbbells-holding hands should be at the side of the head, and the abdominals are tight.
- Slowly lift the dumbbells until the arms are straight. Pause for two seconds.
- Then with the same level of control, return to the starting position with control.
- Repeat this exercise 5 times, rest, and then go for 2 more sets.

Level up: Switch to heavier dumbbells.

Precautions

- Only raise your arms as high as comfortable.
- Keep your core tight.

The Hand Grip

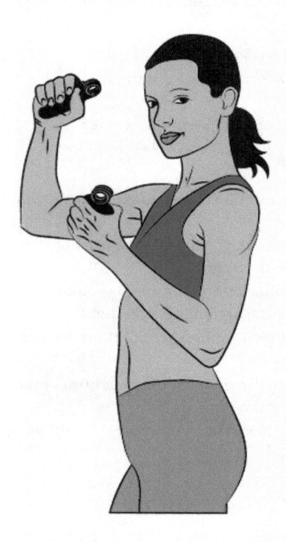

26. Hand Grip

Usually, your grip strength tends to decrease as you age. Thus, this exercise is specifically designed to increase your grip strength, dexterity, and flexibility in your hands and fingers. The hand grip movement can make it easier for you to open door knobs and hold things without dropping them. It is very safe for seniors of any age and grip strength level.

- Other Targeted Areas: Forearms
- Length of workout: 6 mins
- Time durations for resting periods: 10 - 20 secs in-between each set
- Estimated calories burnt: 21 calories.

Instructions

- Grip a soft stress ball in your palm and squeeze it as hard as you can comfortably.
- Hold for 5 -10 seconds and then release.
- Complete 3 sets of 5 to 10 reps on each hand.

Level up: To add intensity, you can switch to using a firmer stress ball when using the soft stress ball becomes easier.

Precautions

- Make sure you warm up your hands before exercising them. This is because this hand grip exercise can lead to finger and wrist strain if the muscles aren't stretched first.
- Totally avoid this exercise if your thumb joint is damaged.

Modified Skull Crusher

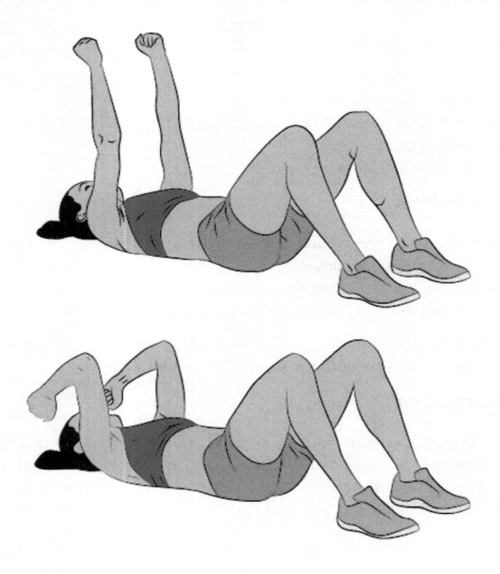

27. Skull Crusher

The skull crusher movement is an isolation exercise that targets and builds your triceps muscle group. It also helps in fixing imbalances with the triceps without you having to place pressure on your wrists. Just so you know, the name "skull crusher" originates from the fact that if you use poor form, you could endanger your skull. Hence you have to be extra careful with it.

- Other Targeted Areas: Upper Arms.
- Length of workout: 7 mins
- Time duration for resting periods: 30 - 40 secs in-between each set.
- Estimated Calories burnt: 27 calories.

Instructions

- Get a flat gym bench and lie on it with your face up and your legs comfortably placed to each side on the floor.
- Hold the dumbbell tight and straight up with both hands above your chest and the dumbbell shaft in a vertical position. Make sure your elbows are not locked.
- Now inhale and slowly move the weight down toward the rear of your head by flexing your elbows while exhaling.
- Only elbows should be moving here, so keep your upper arms from moving back and forth with the weight.
- Continue to lower the weight behind your head until the dumbbell head is about in line with the bench top.
- Slowly reverse the movement to the point where the weight is held above the chest. And you've just completed one rep!
- Repeat 5 to 8 times for each of two sets.

Level up: If you're up for a challenge, try performing this same movement on an inclined bench.

Precautions

- Your starting position should be stable and comfortable.
- Don't lower the weight toward the face or forehead. Instead, ensure that it passes over your head
- Take care not to hit the back of your head when raising the dumbbell from behind the head to return to the starting position.
- This exercise should be done slowly and carefully under good control.

Forward Punches- Warm-Up

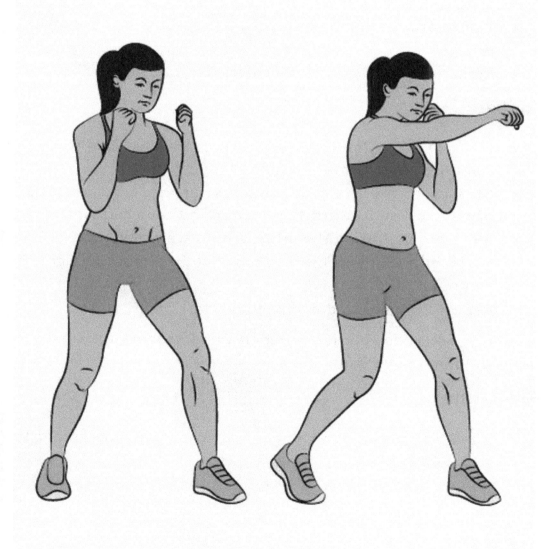

28. Forward Punches

This is a warm-up exercise that you can use to strengthen your shoulder and arms,

- Other targeted areas: Arms
- Length of workout: 10 mins
- Time duration for resting periods: 20-30 secs in-between sets.
- Estimated calorie burn: 59 calories.

Instructions

- Get seated and make fists with your hands. Hold them in front of your chest at shoulder height.
- Envision a punching bag out just at arm's length. Then bring one arm forward to punch it and then return it.
- Alternate and bring the other arm forward and return.
- Make sure that you keep your abdominal muscles tight as you punch.
- Repeat 20 times and complete 5 sets.

Level up: Use water bottles or small hand weights to make the workout more challenging.

Precaution

- Ensure that you don't punch extremely hard so as not to get problems in your upper arms.

Diagonal Shoulder Raise

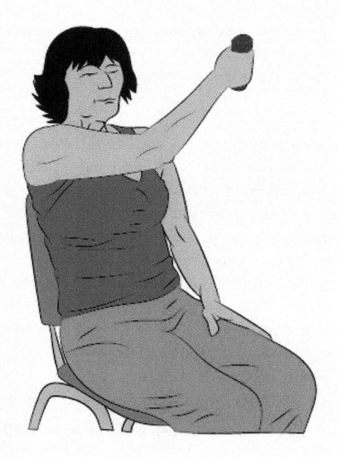

29. Diagonal Shoulder Raise

This shoulder strengthening exercise is a multi-beneficial one for seniors. It helps to improve your shoulder muscle size, function, and neural control. It is also a great tool for fighting and defeating osteoporosis.

- Other targeted areas: Arms
- Length of workout: 5 mins
- Time duration for resting periods: 10 -20 secs in-between sets.
- Estimated calorie burn: 45 calories.

Instructions

- First, sit with a dumbbell in your hand. Your hand should be over your opposite hip with your palm facing inward.
- Next, lift your arm up and across your body to the side. By this time, your palm should be outward.
- Then go back to the start position and do ten repetitions. That's the Diagonal Outwards Shoulder Raise.
- For the inward movement, your palm should be forward,
- Now lift your arm up and across your body to the opposite shoulder. Bend your elbow as you bring your arm over and face your palm inward. Repeat ten times.
- Switch to your other arm and do the same.
- Take a rest and then go for one more set on each hand.

Level up: Switch to heavier weights when you can perform 20 reps easily.

Precautions

- Avoid over-bending your elbows.
- Keep the movements slow.

Chest & Back

Chest Squeeze with Med Ball

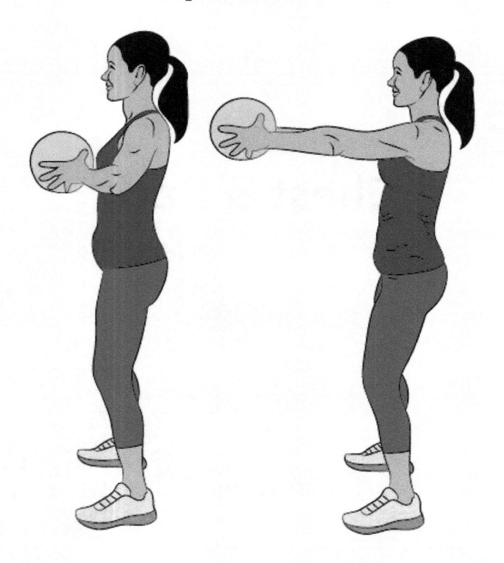

30. Chest Squeeze with Med Ball

At this point, you will notice that the exercises are getting more intense. But trust me, they are still totally easy and fun for seniors of varying fitness levels. This chest squeeze movement is excellent for building and strengthening your chest muscles. Essentially, you're going to need a medicine ball for this to help improve your balance and stability. If you're a beginner in this game, then a good starting point will be around 6 – 8 lbs for older females and 8 -15 lbs for older males.

- Other targeted areas: Arms and glutes.
- Length of workout: 5 mins
- Time duration for resting periods: 20 – 30 secs in-between sets.
- Estimated calorie burn: 48 calories.

Instructions

- Get seated in a sturdy chair with your back straight and feet flat on the floor.
- Tighten your core as you hold the ball with both hands.
- Lift your arms to your chest level by making your elbows bent and out to the sides. Your forearms should be parallel to the floor.
- While putting even tension on the ball with both hands, and squeezing your chest, push the ball forward till your elbows and arms are completely straightened.
- Then pull the ball back to your chest, by bending your elbows.
- Complete 3 sets of 5 reps; resting when necessary.

Level up: To make it more intense, you can wrap a resistance band around your back, with your thumbs/palms at each end of it as you push and pull the medicine ball at your chest level.

Precautions

- Try not to use the Med Ball to hit your chest.
- Use the appropriate weight for your strength level.

Floor Back Extension

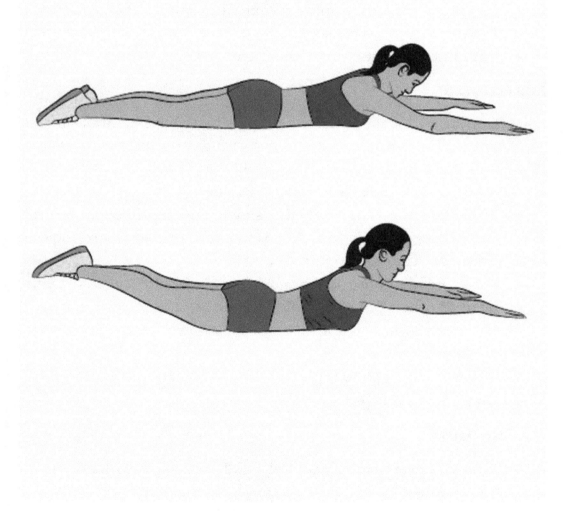

31. Cat and Camel/Floor Back Extension

This is a beginner's stretch that you as a senior will be able to do relatively easily. The cat and camel movement stretch and strengthens your back and abdominal muscles. Thus, giving you the chance to regain or improve your ability to turn and maneuver in your daily activities without the fear of losing your balance.

- Other targeted areas: Abdominal muscles, hips.
- Length of workout: 4 mins x Time duration for resting periods: 5-10secs in-between sets.
- Estimated calorie burn: 20 calories.

Instructions

- Get on all fours, either on a yoga mat, bed, or another soft surface, with your back straight, hands shoulder-width apart, and your fingers facing forward. Your back should also be straight and knees a few inches apart.
- While keeping your abs tight, slowly and gently begin to arch your back and lift your head so that your eyes are looking upwards. That's the cat pose.
- For the camel pose, curve your back upward and lower your head downward. You should feel the stretch in your spine.
- Breathe in when you arch your back down and exhale as you curve your back up.
- That's one complete rep
- Do 2 sets of 5 reps.

Precaution

- Stop the exercise immediately and you begin to feel pain in your spine.

Renegade Arm Row

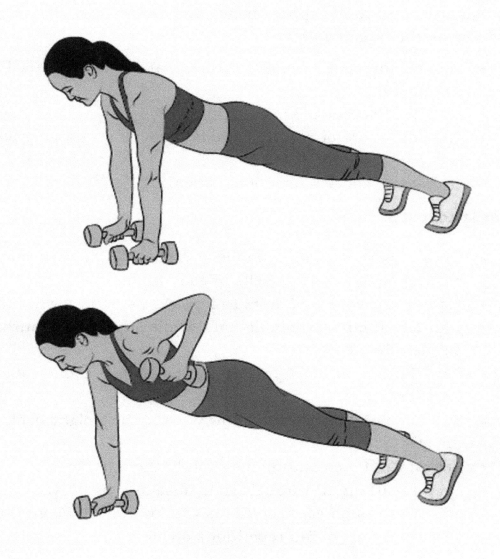

32. Renegade Arm Row

This exercise is an upgrade from the bent-over row and upright row. It targets almost every part of your upper body as well as your core. The renegade arm row also highlights any imbalances in your upper body and eventually helps in stabilizing the targeted areas.

- Other targeted areas: Arms, abdominal muscles, shoulders.
- Length of workout: 8 mins
- Time duration for resting periods: 30 – 60 secs in-between sets.
- Estimated calorie burn: 56 calories.

Instructions

- Grab a pair of light dumbbells and get into a press-up position with the dumbbells in each hand.
- Tighten up your abdominal muscles, as you slowly raise your left dumbbell-holding hand while supporting yourself on the other arm.
- Row the dumbbells upwards till it reaches slightly above your torso.
- Still keeping that control, slowly lower the weight back to the ground.
- Repeat 5-6 times and then switch to the other side.
- Keep breathing in through your nose as you lift your arm and out through your mouth as you lower it to the ground.
- Perform 3 reps of 5-6 repetitions on each side.

Level up: Switch to a heavier weight when you are sure you are ready for the challenge.

Precaution

- Opt. for a lighter dumbbell that is fit for your strength level. Do not overestimate.
- Keep your movement slow and steady.
- It is okay if you cannot raise the dumbbells above your torso; just make sure you go only as high as comfortable.

Bench Press

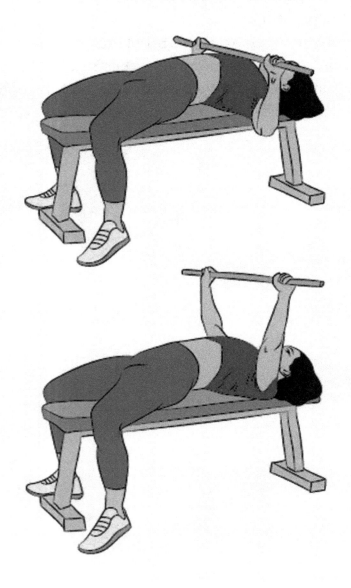

33. Dumbbell Bench Press

This superb compound movement works on your chest muscles to help build enough muscular Strength there. For the fact that it doesn't really require balance, the bench press exercise is one of the safest exercises for seniors especially those with knee problems. However, it is not recommended for those with shoulder pains.

- Other targeted areas: Shoulders, Triceps and Biceps.
- Length of workout: 15 mins
- Time duration for resting periods: 3 minutes in-between each set.
- Estimated calorie burn: 111 calories

Instructions

- Choose a dumbbell that is heavy enough for you to do 12 – 15 reps comfortably but not too comfortably
- Now, lie flat on your back; on a bench, with your feet flat on the ground.
- With a dumbbell in each hand, slowly extend your arms directly above your shoulders, palms facing toward your feet.
- To lower the weights down, squeeze your shoulder blades together and slowly bend your elbows until it is parallel with your shoulders, forming 90-degree angles.
- With the same controlled slow motion, drive the dumbbells back up to start, making sure to squeeze your shoulder blades the entire time. And you have one complete rep!
- Repeat for five to six reps, performing three sets afterward.

Level up: If you're sure that you are fit to take it up a notch, then try the bench press with an Olympic unloaded bar or seated chest machine.

Precautions

- Don't over-squeeze your shoulder blades.
- Rushing with your movement will only increase your injury risk so do them slowly.

Mid-Back Extension

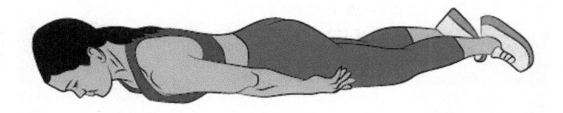

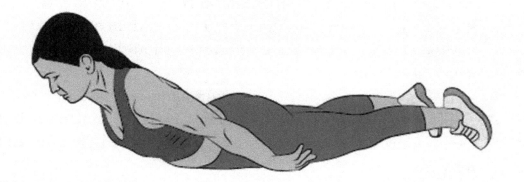

34. Mid-Back Extension

This exercise is also known as the prone cobra movement. It basically focuses on stretching, extending, and strengthening your lower back and mid-back muscles, making it easier for you to maintain good posture when sitting or standing. It can also help to relieve mid back pain associated with postural strain.

- Other targeted areas: Neck, Arms
- Length of workout: 7 mins
- Time duration for resting periods: 30 – 40 secs in between each set
- Estimated calorie burn: 32 calories

Instructions

- Start by lying face down on your bed or the floor with your hand and palm down by the side of your face. For comfort, you may place your forehead on a rolled-up hand towel.
- Slowly pinch your shoulder blades together and lift your hands off the floor. Your shoulder should be down and away from ears
- Roll your elbows in with your palms out and thumbs up.
- Gently lift your forehead about an inch off the towel but keep your eyes looking straight at the floor and not forward.
- Try to hold that position for 10 seconds.
- Make sure that you maintain your hips on the floor and don't hold your breath. Keep breathing in through your nose and out through your mouth.
- Return to the starting position and repeat 5 times. Take a rest and go for two more sets.

Level up: To increase the intensity of the exercise slightly, you can also lift your legs off the ground.

Precautions

- Keep your movement very slow and controlled

Reverse Flyers

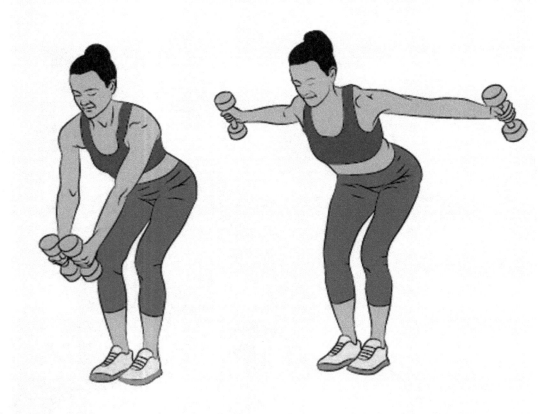

35. Reverse Flyers

The reverse fly is a resistance exercise that targets the major muscles of the upper back, including the trapezius. This exercise helps to improve your stamina by strengthening these muscles that are usually negatively affected by poor posture.

- Other targeted areas: Neck, Rear shoulders, and upper back
- Length of workout: 10 mins
- Time duration for resting periods: 30 – 40 secs in-between each set.
- Estimated calorie burn: 36 calories.

Instructions

- Stand upright with your arms holding dumbbells at the sides and feet shoulder-width apart
- Slowly, press your hips back in a hinge motion bringing your chest forward almost parallel to the floor.
- Allow the weights to hang straight down, as you maintain a tight core, straight back, and slight knee bend.
- Breathe out and raise both arms out to your side, squeezing the shoulder blades together.
- Bend your elbows a little bit as you pull your shoulder blades toward the spine. x Now, take in a deep breath as you lower the weight back to the starting position.
- Avoid hunching your shoulders up during the movement, instead, keep your chin tucked and focus on feeling the shoulders blades coming together.
- Repeat the exercise for 4 times for 3 sets.

Level up: Increase weight resistance during the exercise by lifting heavier dumbbells.

Precautions

- Don't ignore the breathing rules.
- Keep your shoulder back throughout the movement.

Hips

Lying Hip Bridges

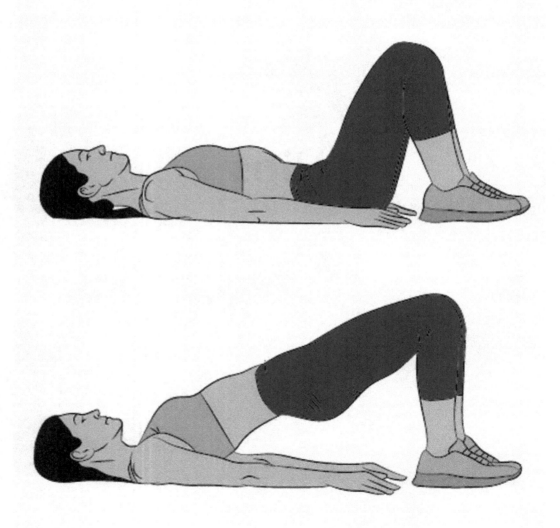

36. Lying Hip Bridges

Lying hip bridges is one of the most important strength-training hips exercises for seniors. It targets and works your body's largest muscle group, which is the glutes; your butt muscles. Fortunately, it starts and ends with you lying on your back.

- Other targeted areas: Abs, hamstrings, lower back
- Length of workout: 7 mins
- Time duration for resting periods: 20 - 30 in-between each set.
- Estimated calorie burn: 32 calories

Instructions

- Lie on your back with your hands by your side, knees bent, and feet flat on the floor.
- Flatten your lower back against the floor, to tighten your abdominals and squeeze your butt muscles, then lift your hips into the air to create a straight line from your knees to shoulders.
- As you lift your hips, push through your feet.
- Hold for 10 to 15 seconds, and then slowly lower your hips and return to your starting position.
- Complete 2-3 sets of 10 reps.

Level up: Use a resistance band to bind your legs and follow these same instructions. You will surely find it more intense.

Precautions

- Lower your back to the ground once you begin to feel pain. You don't have to hold the hip bridge pose for up to 15 seconds.

Side Hip Raise

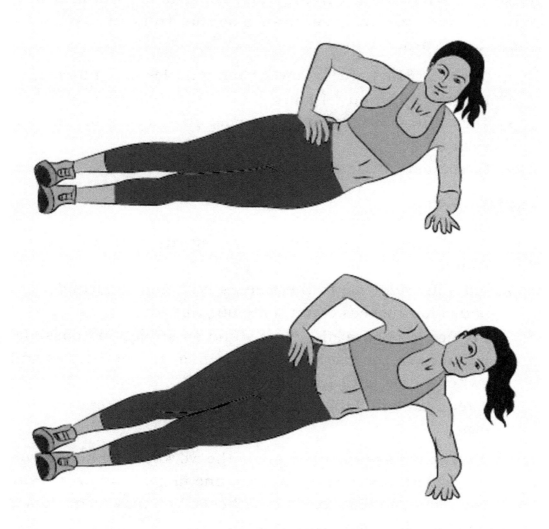

37. Side hip raise

The exercise is an exceptional hip arthritis-relieving exercise that delivers great results for seniors and the elderly. It minimizes your pains and safely strengthens your side hip muscles. Performing it correctly and consistently will also help improve your lower body endurance so that you can easily walk and sidestep around objects.

- Other targeted areas: Lower back muscles and glutes.
- Length of workout: 4 mins
- Time duration for resting periods: 10 -20 secs in-between each set.
- Estimated calorie burn: 25 calories.

Instructions

- Stand upright and hold on to a sturdy chair to balance yourself.
- Lift your right leg to the side as high as comfortable and pause for a 2 secs count. Lift your ribs too!
- Try not to bend at the hips; stand as straight as possible. x Return to the starting position, then repeat 5 times and switch to the left leg.
- After completing that, go for one more set of 5 reps on both legs.

Level up: To increase the intensity of the workout, try holding on to the chair with just one hand, then one finger, and eventually let go completely to balance on your heels. You may also add a 2 to 5-pound ankle weight to your leg.

Precautions

- Keep your body erect and breathe properly
- Don't lift your hips too high.

Pelvic Tilt

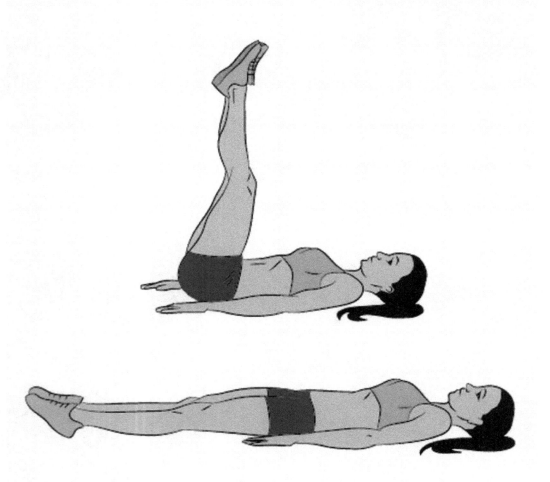

38. Pelvic Tilt

The pelvic tilt exercise is a stretch and strength-building movement combined. It is beneficial for releasing tight hips caused by prolonged sitting. It also helps to increase the range of motion and flexibility of the pelvic region.

- Other targeted areas: Core and lower back.
- Length of workout: 6 mins x Time duration for resting periods: 30 seconds to a minute between each set.
- Estimated calorie burn: 25 calories.

Instructions

- Lie on your back, whether on your mat or bed with your knees bent and feet flat on the ground.
- Tightening abdominal muscles, push your lower back into the floor. Release a deep breath while letting your hips and pelvis also rock back.
- Hold this position for five seconds, then relax with your lower back rising off the ground slightly.
- Make sure to inhale as you relax.
- Repeat 2-3 sets of 5 reps.

Level up: Combine this pelvic tilt exercise with alternating arm raises to take it up a notch!

Precaution

- Keep your spine straight as you lower your back

Hip Extensions

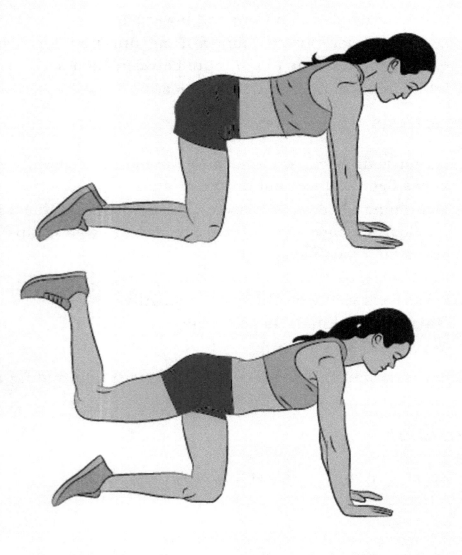

39. Hip Extensions

These hip extension exercises target and strengthen your legs, and hip flexor muscles. Strengthening these muscles will, in turn, improve your balance and assist in walking and standing. Before you know it, you will be propelling yourself forward or up the stairs easily and without any help.

- Other targeted areas: Glutes, hamstrings.
- Length of workout: 4 mins
- Time duration for resting periods: 10 -20 secs in-between each set.
- Estimated calorie burn: 25 calories

Instructions

- Stand upright, using a chair to balance yourself.
- Tighten your tummy muscles and keep breathing as you slowly extend your left leg backward. Keep your body erect and your knee straight.
- Pause a little, then gently lower your leg back to the ground to return to the start position
- Repeat 2 sets of 10 reps with each leg.

Level up: For a more challenging workout, add a 2 to 5-pound weight to your ankles. But first, try using a single hand, one finger, or no hands to balance yourself.

Precautions

- If you have knee problems, use two chairs instead of one for support.

Hip Abductions

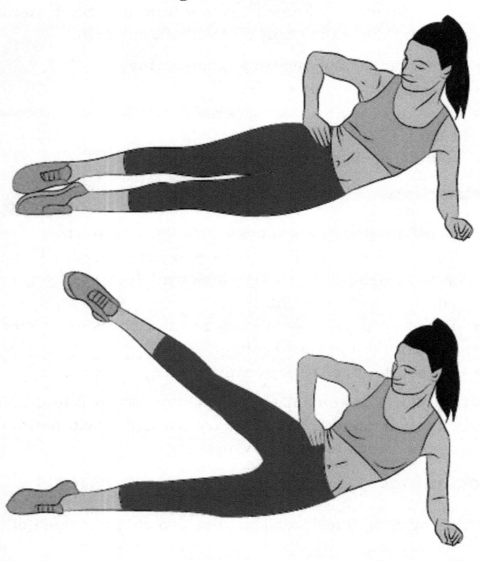

40. Hip Abductions

This exercise aims to build and strengthen your hip abductors. It also trains your lower body to provide core stability, build balance, and good posture.

- Other targeted areas: abdominals, back muscles, buttocks (glutes).
- Length of workout: 5 mins
- Time duration for resting periods: 20 - 30 secs in-between sets
- Estimated calorie burn: 29 calories.

Instructions

- Standing tall with your feet close together and hold on to a sturdy chair.
- Your hip, knee, and foot should be pointing straight forward with your body erect x Slowly lift your leg out to the side and in a controlled motion bringing your feet back together.
- Pause for 3-5 secs. Make sure that you do not lean or hitch your pelvis during this pose.
- Gently return to the starting position.
- Repeat for 2-3 sets of 4 repetitions on each leg.

Level up: Place a resistance band around both your legs at the thigh level.

Precautions

Try not to hitch your pelvic throughout the movement.

Never hold your breath.

Baz Thompson

Knees

Knee Extension

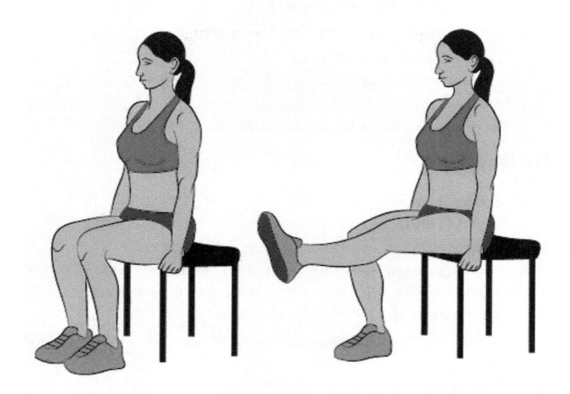

41. Knee Extension

The ability to stand easily and fully extend your knee is very vital for every human being. Unfortunately, aging causes the knee joints to lose some of their flexibility and range of motion. That's why this knee extension exercise aims to strengthen your knee joints, thus improving your ability to stand and balance as well as your available knee range of motion.

- Other targeted areas: Quadriceps (Thighs)
- Length of workout: 6 mins
- Time duration for resting periods: 30 - 40 secs in-between each set.
- Estimated calorie burn: 31 calories.

Instructions

- Sit up tall in a chair with your feet flat on the floor and your shoulders back and down.
- Slowly lift your leg up and extend the knee.
- Hold for a few seconds when you have fully straightened that knee. At the same time, try squeezing the muscles at the front of the thigh.
- Next, slowly lower your leg back down and alternate your legs.
- To use your full range of motion, ensure to bring your heel fully back as far as comfortable then extend.
- Repeat for 3 sets of 5 reps and rest where necessary

Level up: To take this exercise a step higher and accelerate your strengthening, add ankle weights to your ankle.

Precautions

- Using immense control, move your leg slowly without jerking it.
- Do not hold your breath. Inhale as you lift your leg and exhale as you lower it back to the ground.
- Your back should remain straight against the chair, so no slouching!

Squat Curl Knee Lift

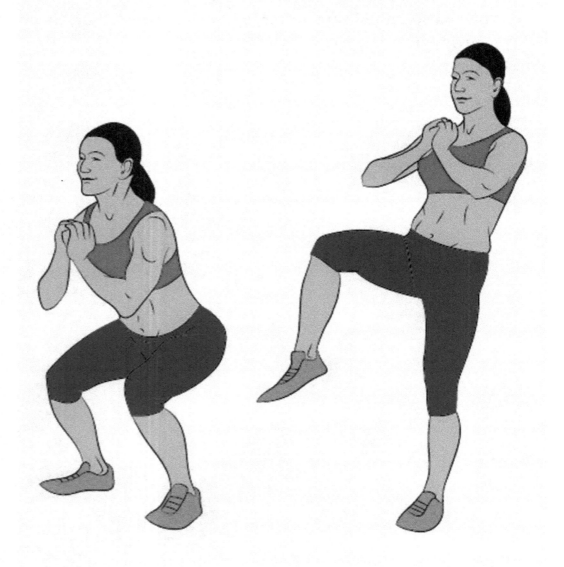

42. Squat Curl Knee Lift

Of course, the combination of three individual exercises into one will definitely seem intimidating if not totally impossible especially for seniors. But you don't have any cause to worry since the squat, curl and knee lift movements are all super basic and easy to learn if you haven't tried them out already. This multitasking strength training exercise works a lot of different muscles all at once with a major focus on your knees and quads. It is also a very reliable way to help lessen the symptoms of the following chronic conditions like arthritis and osteoporosis. Another great thing is that all you need is a pair of dumbbells.

- Other targeted areas: biceps, glutes, quads.
- Length of workout: 10 mins x Time duration for resting periods: 30 secs - 1 minute in-between each set.
- Estimated calorie burn: 28 calories.

Instructions

- Start in a squat position with your chest lifted, shoulders down, and abs tight.
- Weight back on your heels with your arms straight next to your side, holding dumbbells.
- Squeeze your glutes to press upwards and lift your right knee as you curl the weights to your shoulders.
- When you curl, ensure that your elbows are as close to your body as you can.
- Now, lower the dumbbells back down and return to your squat position. Then repeat with the left knee.
- Perform 2-3 sets of 5 reps per side.

Level up: Switch to heavier dumbbells.

Precautions

- Make sure to choose weights that can create enough resistance for your biceps to feel the burn. However, ensure that it is not at the expense of you losing your form or feel any form of pain.
- Do not rush with this movement; just keep your movement slow and well-controlled.
- Do not let your knees go over the toes too far as that can place excessive pressure on your knee joints.

Knee Curl

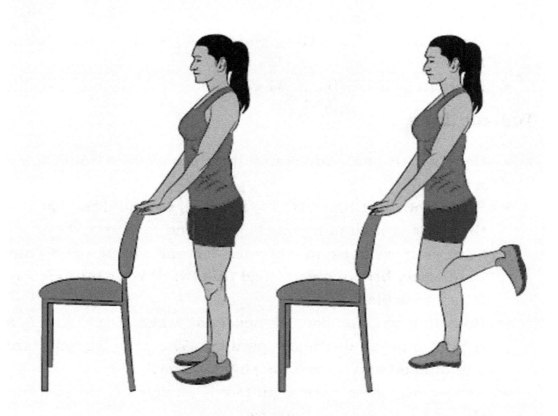

43. Knee Curl

This exercise is an ideal exercise for you as a senior to improve your leg strength and balance. Kneel curls strengthen your hamstring muscles and having stronger hamstrings, in turn, helps in strengthening your knee joints. It also improves their flexibility and balancing abilities

- Other targeted areas: Hamstring muscles x Length of workout: 10 minutes.
- Time duration for resting periods: 40 secs - 1-minute in-between sets.
- Estimated calorie burn: 31 calories.

Instructions

- Get a sturdy chair and stand upright with your front-facing it.
- Space your feet hip-distance apart as you hold the back of the chair to maintain your balance and for support.
- Shift your weight onto your left leg and slowly bend your right knee, bringing your heel up toward your buttocks as far as possible.
- Hold this position for 1-3 seconds. Make sure your hips remain still and thighs parallel. The left leg you are standing on should also be slightly bent.
- Now, slowly lower your right foot back down to the ground. Go for 8 - 10 reps on your right leg.
- Then switch to your other leg for the same amount of reps. This will complete one set. Aim for 2-3 sets.

Level up: If you're up for a challenge, perform the same motions without holding the back of the chair for balance.

Precautions

- Ensure that you do not arch your back as you lower and lift your leg.
- Keep your movements slow and controlled without any jerks. Rushing will only result in injury.

Knee Thrusters

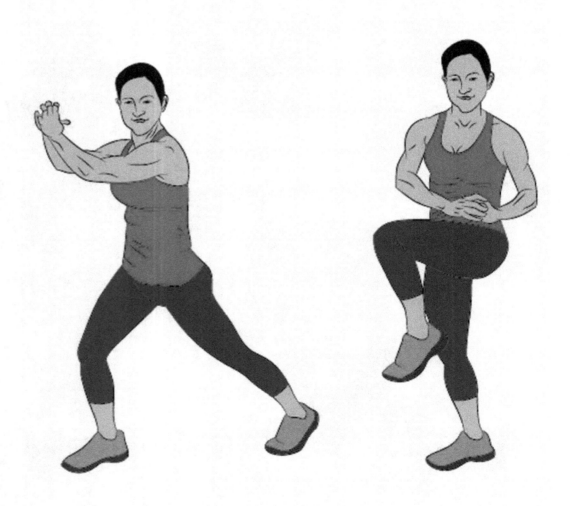

44. Knee Thrusters

Knee thrusters are great low-impact exercises that strengthen your lower body and core while getting your heart rate up. This in turn helps in improving your pelvic stability. The idea here is that you're visually crushing something against your knee

- Other targeted areas: hip flexors, back muscles, core (abdominals), triceps, shoulders
- Length of workout: 5 mins
- Time duration for resting periods: 20 -30 secs in-between each set.
- Estimated calorie burn: 25 calories.

Instructions

- Get into a standing position with your feet wider than shoulder-distance apart.
- Turn both feet in one direction, allowing your hips to follow in the same direction like you're doing a shallow lunge.
- The front knee should be at a 90-degree angle with the back heel lifted. Also, extend your arms up in a guard position in front of the chest.
- Lift your back knee up to your hip height toward the hands, then lower your hands in toward the thigh.
- Return the foot to the floor. Repeat 6-8 times and then alternate legs.
- Complete 2-3 sets of 6-8 reps on each leg.

Level up: To add more resistance, you can use a resistance band around your knees.

Precautions

- Keep your movement slow, controlled and smooth.

Knee Lift with Med Ball

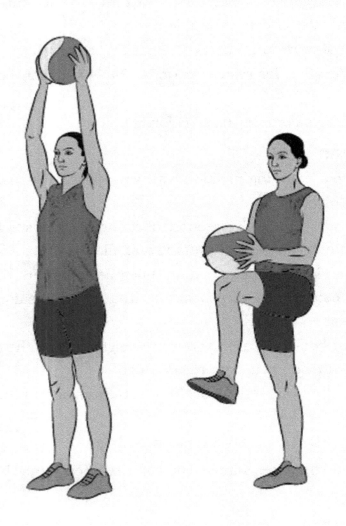

45. Hip Marching

The hip marching exercise is designed to strengthen your hips and knees. By doing this, this movement also improves your walking endurance and ability to bend pick up objects off lower surfaces.

- Other targeted areas: thighs, abdominal muscles.
- Length of workout: 7 mins
- Time duration for resting periods: 30 -40 secs in-between each set
- Estimated calorie burn: 21 calories

Instructions

- Sit in a chair with your feet flat on the floor and your back straight against your back.
- Slowly, lift up your right knee as high as comfortable.
- Hold the position for one second and then gently lower your leg.
- Alternate lifting your knees for 5 reps on each leg, then rest and go for one more set.

Level up: Place your hands on your thighs and resist the upward movement of your knees by pushing downward.

Precautions

- Move at a slow to moderate speed and continue breathing throughout the exercise.
- No matter how strong you might feel, don't perform more than 20 hip-marching moves in a row. That is your best option to avoid fatigue and soreness.

Baz Thompson

Ankle and Feet

Chair Stand

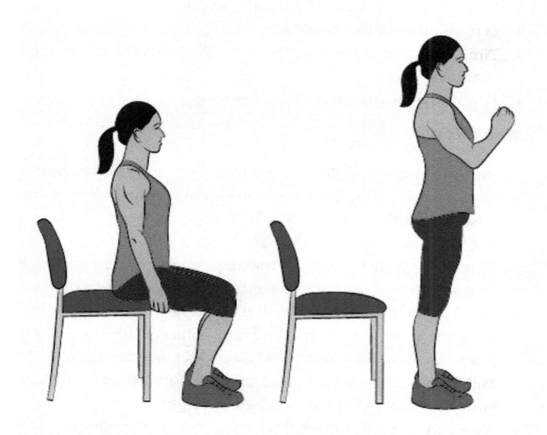

46. Chair Stands

This exercise helps in increasing your leg strength with major focus on your ankles and feet. By doing this, the chair stand movement also improves your balance, standing stamina as well as body posture.

- Other Targeted Areas: Back, abs and thighs.
- Length of workout: 6 mins
- Time duration for resting periods: 20 -30 secs in-between each set.
- Estimated calories burnt: 19 calories.

Instructions

- Sit toward the middle or edge of an armless sturdy chair.
- Then slightly lean back so that you are in a half-reclining position, with your back and shoulders straight, knees bent, and feet flat on the floor.
- Now using your hands as little as possible, bring your back forward so that you are now sitting in an upright position.
- Keeping your back straight and drawing in your abdominal muscles, slowly stand up, using your hands as little as possible again. You should take at least 3 seconds to stand up.
- Make sure that as you bend slightly forward to stand up, your back and shoulders remain straight.
- When you have fully stood in a upright position, take another 3 seconds to sit back down. That's one rep.
- Complete 2 sets of 8 to 15 reps, taking rest when necessary.

Level up: As you become stronger, try doing this exercise without using your hands.

Precautions

- Every of your movements should be slow and steady.
- Keep back and shoulders straight throughout exercise.
- If you're finding it difficult to keep your back straight on your own, try placing pillows against the lower back of the chair first, for support.

Toe Stand

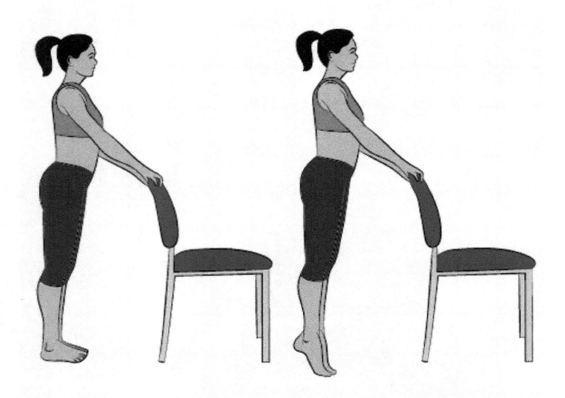

47. Toe Stand

Toe stand are another leg strengthening exercise that targets your toes and the muscles in the front of your legs. It also helps you strengthen your balance and flexibility abilities.

- Other targeted areas: Leg muscles,
- Length of workout: 7 mins
- Time duration for resting periods: 10 – 20 secs in-between each set.
- Estimated calorie burn: 19 calories

Instructions

- Start seated with your back straight and both feet firmly planted on the ground.
- Slowly, lift your toes off the floor as high as you can. You should feel the stretch in your toe as you hold that position for 3-5 seconds.
- Then lower your toes back down to the floor. Do 3 sets of 10 reps.

Level up: Perform the same number of reps while standing. You might want to consider using a sturdy chair for support at first. Then go-ahead to try standing on your own.

Precautions

- Of course, you should feel a stretch in your toes during these movements. However, do not confuse that with pain. The moment you start to feel pain, take a break!
- Do not arch your back.

Rest of the Lower Body

Chair Squat

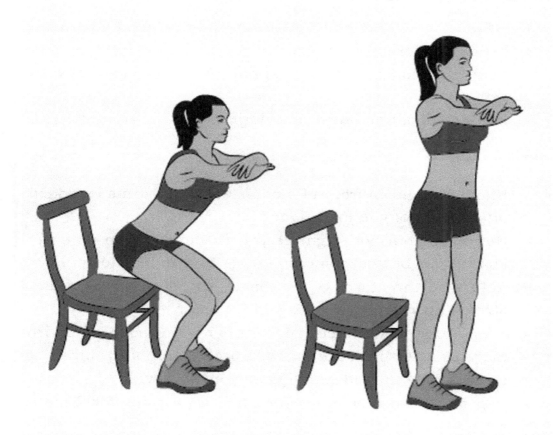

48. Chair Squat

The chair squat saves you from the intense stress of the standard squat movement and at the same time, it ensures that you don't miss out on any benefit. With the safety of a sturdy chair, you get to strengthen and stabilize your leg muscles without the fear of falling.

- Other targeted areas: Hamstrings, quadriceps, and glutes.
- Length of workout: 6 mins
- Time duration for resting periods: 20-30 secs in-between sets.
- Estimated calorie burn: 31 calories

Instructions

- Stand straight in front of a chair with your arms extended out in front of you for balance.
- Now keep your core tight as you slowly sit down onto the chair. Your buttocks should be the first to hit the chair.
- Return to the starting position by standing back up and stretching your arms out again for balance.
- Keep your back nice and straight during the entire movement. Also ensure that you breathe properly, inhaling as you come up and exhaling as you sit down.
- Repeat 10 times before resting and then going for 2 more sets.

Level up: Replace your empty extended hands with dumbbells that are fit for your strength level.

Precautions

- A recliner or a bar stool height chair is a total No-No!.
- Use a sturdy chair that is the proper height for you.
- Pay close attention to your form and make sure you are doing it right. This will help minimize stress on your back.

Hamstring Curl

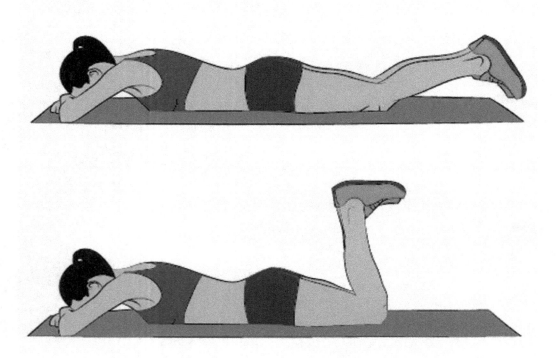

49. Hamstring Curls

Being able to balance your hamstrings, which are the muscles located on the back of the thighs, is essential for walking and standing abilities. However, aging has the potential of taking that ability from you. Fortunately, the hamstring curl is another effective exercise that will improve the balance, flexibility, and range of motion of your hamstrings. This will in turn decrease your likelihood of falls and risks of injury in that area.

- Other targeted areas: upper and lower back muscles.
- Length of workout: 10 mins
- Time duration for resting periods: 40 secs – 1 minute in-between each set.
- Estimated calorie burn: 35 calories

Instructions

- Get seated in a chair with your feet flat on the ground.
- Slowly, extend your left leg up slightly and position your left heel on the floor.
- Now lean forward at the hips and reach toward your left toes.
- Hold the stretch for 10 – 20 secs. No doubt, you will surely feel a stretch in your hamstrings.
- Sit back up and return your leg and arm to the starting position.
- Repeat 10 times before switching to your right leg and doing the same amount of reps.
- Relax a little and then go for one more set of 10 reps on each leg

Level up: If you are sure and ready to take this exercise a notch up, try doing the same movement while standing up straight. The only difference here is that you will be bending forward at the waist and reaching towards your toes.

Precautions

- Stop immediately if you experience any pain or extreme discomfort. The best thing to do is to either readjust your position, reduce your range of motion or take a break until the pain subsides.

The Chair Dip

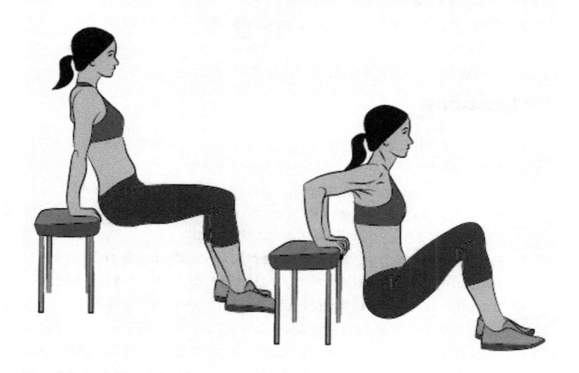

50. The Chair Dip

Chair dips are strength-training exercises that are not just simple and effective, but also very easy to incorporate into your routine. Basically, this exercise targets the muscles on the back of the upper arms as well as your lower body.

- Other targeted areas: Triceps.
- Length of workout: 7 mins
- Time duration for resting periods: 30 – 40 secs in-between each set
- Estimated calorie burn: 32 calories

Instructions

- Sit on your chair with your arms on its armrests and your feet flat on the floor, hip distance apart.
- Your fingers should grip the arms of the chair as you move your torso forward off the chair with your arms fully extended and your knees slightly bent.
- Breathe in as you slowly lower your body back to the seat, hinging at your elbows until they form a 90-degree angle.
- Exhale as you push up back to your starting position with your arms fully extended.
- Complete 3 sets of 5-10 reps. As you build Strength, you may work your way up to doing more repetitions or sets of the exercise.

Level up: To increase the difficulty of this exercise, completely straighten your legs as you lift your torso. Also, try placing just your heels on the floor instead of the whole foot.

Precautions

- Resist the constant temptation to shrug your shoulders during movement. Try to keep them neutral with your neck in a relaxed position.

Side Leg Raise

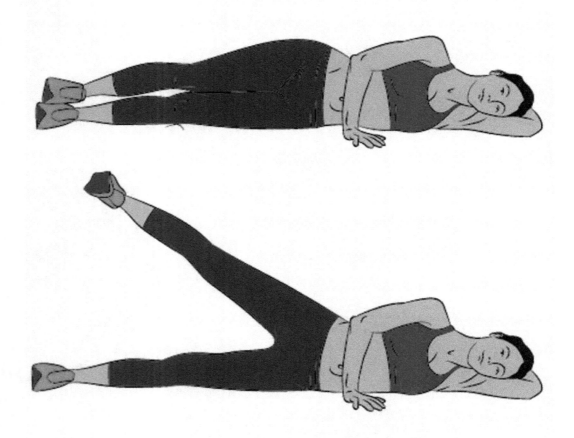

51. Side Leg Raise

Performing side leg raises is an easy and effective way to increase your lower body strength while improving its balance and flexibility abilities simultaneously. Over time, you get to enjoy your increased functional independence with reduced falls and lower injury risks.

- Other targeted areas: lower back muscles, pelvis, quadriceps, and hip flexor.
- Length of workout: 6 mins
- Time duration for resting periods: 10 – 20 secs in-between each set
- Estimated calorie burn: 36 calories.

Instructions

- Stand directly behind or beside the chair with your back straight and your feet flat to the floor slightly apart.
- Hold onto the back of the chair and take a deep breath.
- Now as you exhale, slowly lift your right leg off the floor and extend it out to the side.
- It doesn't matter if it is just 2 or 3 inches. Be sure that it will get better with time.
- Keep your two legs straight as inhale and hold this pose for 5-10 seconds.
- Breathe out as you slowly return to your starting position.
- Repeat 8 times on the right side then switch to the other leg and do the same. That's one set
- Perform 2 more sets.

Level up: Try letting go of the chair or using a comfortable resistance band around your thighs to make this exercise more challenging.

Precautions

- Do not lift your leg too high off the ground.

Back Leg Raise

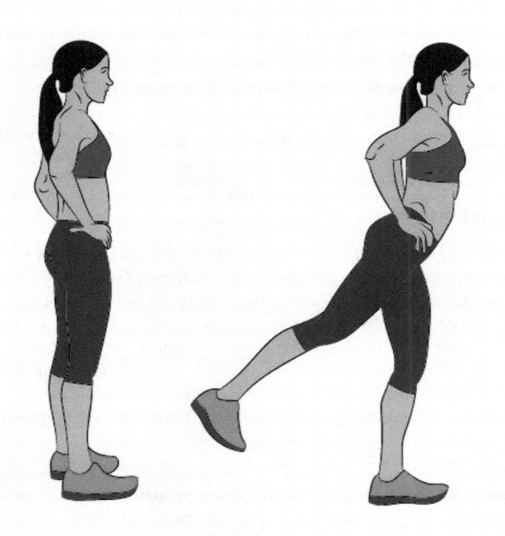

52. Back Leg Raise

This relatively easy-to-perform exercise plays a large role in strengthening your leg and lower body as well as improving your body mobility and balance. Just like the side raises, the back leg raises may require you to have some balance and Strength. So, don't be discouraged if it takes some time to work up to a perfect back leg raise!

- Other targeted areas: lower back muscles and glutes
- Length of workout: 5 mins
- Time duration for resting periods: 10 – 20 secs in-between each set.
- Estimated calorie burn: 25 calories.

Instructions

- Stand up straight with your feet hip-width apart and your hands resting lightly on a chair in front of you.
- Slowly lift your right leg and extend it straight out behind you. Again, it is okay if your leg is just a little bit off the ground. Just make sure you feel comfortable and safe.
- Maintain that position for a count of at least 5 and then gently lower your foot back down to the ground.
- Return your leg to its starting position and repeat with your left leg.
- Do this exercise for 3 sets of 5 reps on each leg.

Level up: Try letting go of the chair or using a comfortable resistance band around your thighs to make this exercise more challenging.

Precautions

- Try as much as possible not to bend your knees.
- Keep your shoulders back and chin up during the entire movement.
- Also, remember to do most of the lifting with your abdominal muscles, so keep your core tight!

Seated Marching On the Spot

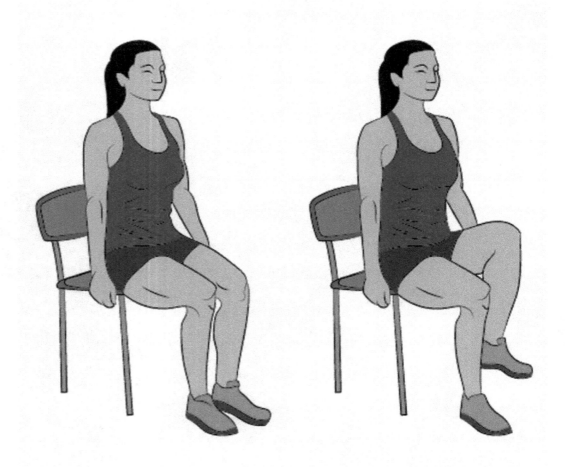

53. Seated Marching on the Spot

Though it is done in a seated position, this exercise involves you constantly moving and contracting your leg muscles which improves muscle strength, stability, and flexibility. Marching on the spot is also a great balance exercise that may help to reduce pain in your knees while making them stronger and healthier.

- Other targeted areas: Hamstrings, glutes, and hip flexors.
- Length of workout: 4 mins
- Time duration for resting periods: 20 – 39 secs in-between each set.
- Estimated calorie burn: 19 calories

Instructions

- Sit upright in a sturdy chair with your spine straight and your feet hip-width apart.
- Slowly, lift your right knee as high as comfortable then gently lower it. Also, lift the left leg and lower it.
- Lift and lower your legs 10 times, then rest and go for 2 more sets.

Level up: Do this movement while standing.

Precautions

- Don't raise your knee too high

Wall Slides

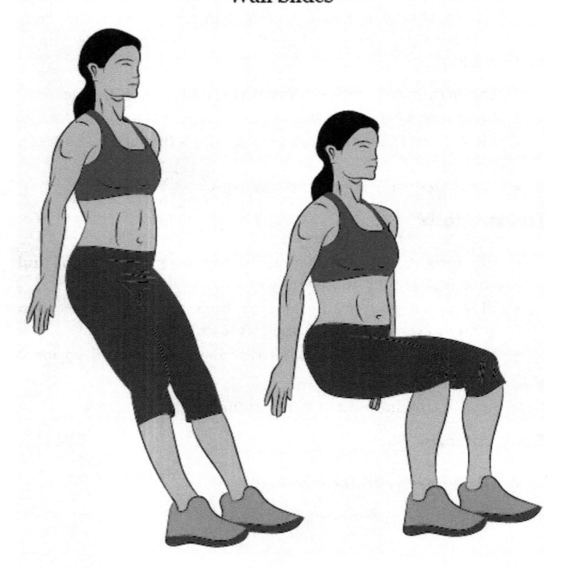

54. Wall Slides

Wall slides are excellent exercises that can help increase the Strength of your major leg muscles with an immense focus on your quads, glutes, and calves. As an elderly person, you can also use the wall slide movement to beat back bad posture and increase your body mobility.

- Other targeted areas: shoulder, neck, and back muscles
- Length of workout: 5 mins
- Time duration for resting periods: 30 -40 secs in-between each set.
- Estimated calorie burn: 31 calories

Instructions

- Begin by standing upright with your back against a wall and your feet shoulder-width apart.
- Still pressing your back and shoulder blades into the wall, bring your arms up.
- The backs of your hands should be against the wall with your thumbs at about the height of your head. The line of your upper arm, from your elbow to shoulder, should also be parallel to the floor.
- Inhale, as you slowly bend your knees and slide your back down the wall until your knees are bent at a 45-degree angle. At the same time, straighten your elbows until your arms are extended straight up over your head. However, still, place it against the wall.
- Hold this position for 5 seconds.

- Exhale as you straighten your knees to slide back up the wall until you are fully standing upright with your knees straight and elbows bent back to their starting position.
- Do 2-3 sets of 5 reps.

Level up: Add dumbbells to the wall slides workout routine.

Precautions

Your bent knees shouldn't go beyond a maximum of a 45-degree angle. Bending more than this will place increased strain on your knees, thus putting yourself at risk for injury.

As you build more Strength and become familiar with this movement, it is very easy for you to lose focus. However, ensure that your movement remains smooth and slow while always checking in your form to confirm if you're doing it correctly.

Full-body

Jog in Place

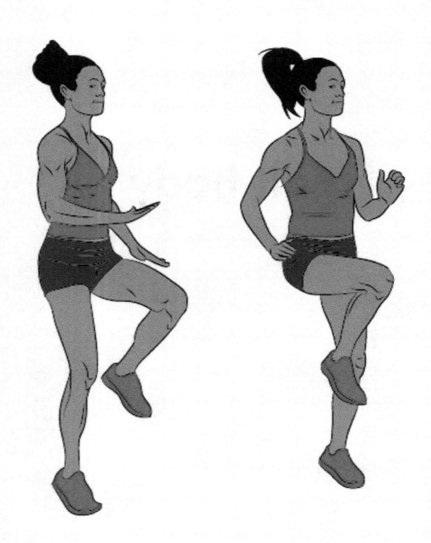

55. Jog in place – warm-up

Considering the needs of an aging body, the Jog in place is an excellent warm-up exercise you can use to get your heart pumping and your body ready before going fully into the more intense strength-training workouts.

- Other targeted areas: calves, quads, and hamstrings.
- Length of workout: 8 mins
- Time duration for resting periods: 50 secs - 1 minute in-between each set
- Estimated calorie burn: 45 calories

Instructions

- Stand up and tall with your feet hip-distance apart.
- Slowly lift one foot up then the other to jog in place.
- Remember to draw in your abdominals as you jog.
- Go for 3 sets of 5 reps resting when necessary.

Level up: To accelerate your full-body strength-training from this exercise, try holding weights that are befitting for your fitness level. Doing this will also help you work your upper body as well.

Precautions

- In case this movement is too much for you, then go for the low-impact movement where you just march with high knees in place.

Bird Dog

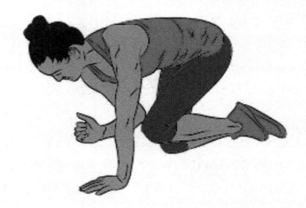

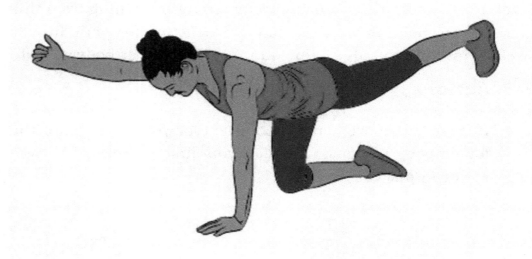

56. Bird Dog

Bird dog is a very simple bodyweight and core exercise that helps in strengthening your core, hips, and back muscles. It can also improve your posture as well as increase the range of motion of its targeted joint areas.

- Other targeted areas: Glutes
- Length of workout: 6 minutes
- Time duration for resting periods: 40 secs - 1 minute in-between each set.
- Estimated calorie burn: 41 calories

Instructions

- Get on all fours; on the mat with your hands underneath your shoulder and your knees bent at 90 degrees directly under your hips.
- Engage your core and exhale as you slowly reach your right arm long.
- While maintaining that position, extend the opposite leg long behind you.
- Hold that position for a second and then slowly lower your leg and arm back to the ground. Remember to inhale as you lower your body.
- Repeat on the left arm and your right leg.
- Perform 3 sets of 5 reps on each side.

Level up: Use a resistance band around your thighs area as you complete these exercises.

Precautions

- This exercise can seem so complicated but it really isn't complex. Just ensure that your movements are slow and steady.
- Keep your back straight!
- Avoid lifting your leg too high because it might cause your spine to curve past its natural position, leading to injury.

Sit to Stand

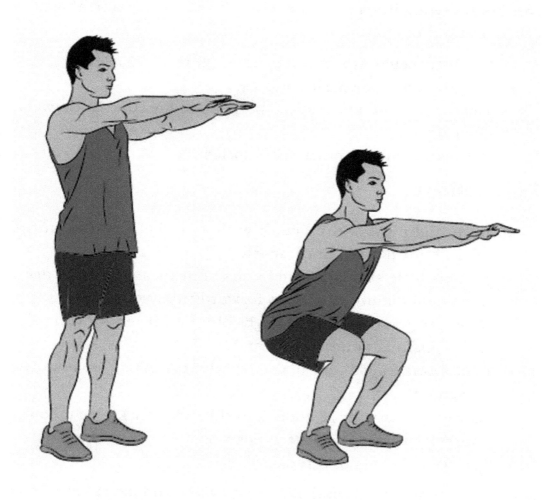

57. Sit to Stand

Sit-and-stands are one of the best legs strengthening exercises for seniors who may struggle with standing up from low chairs or from soft couches. It helps you improve leg strength, functional balance, and control. Eventually, these beneficial uses can restore your independence when it comes to your ability to get in and out of chairs and even walk!

- Other targeted areas: hip flexors, glutes.
- Length of workout: 10 minutes.
- Time duration for resting periods: 1 minute in-between each set.
- Estimated calorie burn: 39 calories.

Instructions

- Sit upright in a sturdy chair with your feet planted on the floor about hip-distance apart.
- With as little support from hands or arms as possible, draw in your abdominals and tip forward from your hips.
- Now, put your weight through all four corners of your feet while pushing yourself to stand.
- Once your knees and hips are fully extended, reverse the movement.
- Slowly, press your hips back and bend your knees to lower yourself back to the seated position.
- Perform 2-3 sets of 6 reps.

Level up: Try holding dumbbells as you raise and lower your body during this exercise

Precautions

- If you can't lift your body all the way to a standing position, simply shift your weight forward and lift your glutes an inch or two from the chair seat.
- Then hold that pose for a second before lowering back down. Over time, you will develop the Strength and balance necessary to rise to a standing position.

Good Mornings

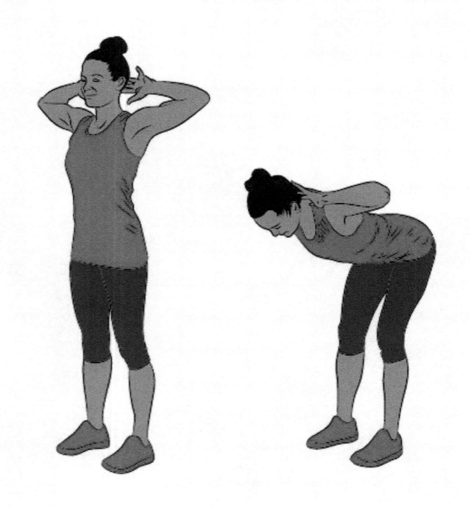

58. Good Mornings

Good mornings are great for improving your back health as a senior. It also helps in strengthening your lower-back muscles and core.

- Other targeted areas: Hamstring, abs.
- Length of workout: 7 mins
- Time duration for resting periods: 20 - 40 secs in-between each set.
- Estimated calorie burn: 32 calories

Instructions

- Stand upright with your feet shoulder-width apart and your hands placed behind your head.
- Brace your core and pull your shoulders back, as you take in a breath and hinge forwards from your hips, not your waist.
- Slightly bend your knees and keep your back flat.
- Then lean forward until you feel a slight stretch in your hamstrings. However, make sure not to go beyond horizontal. Pause a little.
- Exhale and reverse the move to stand up straight.
- Complete 2-3 sets of 6 reps, resting when necessary.

Level up: To make this exercise more intense, stand on a large looped resistance band with both feet and bring the other side of the loop over your head so it rests on your shoulders. Complete the good morning exercise in this position.

Precautions

- Make sure you get the form consistently perfect right through the set before progressing to using a resistance band or barbell with plates.
- Keep the movements slow.

Calf Raises

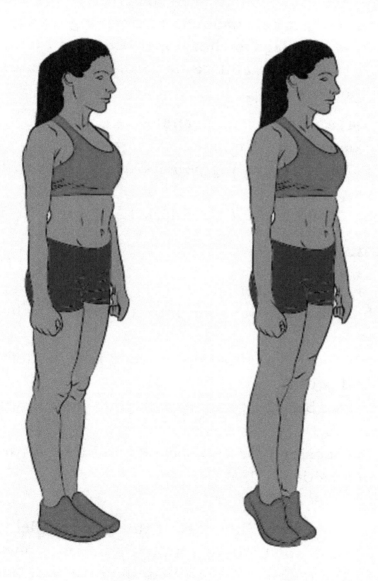

59. Calf Raises

Strengthening your calf muscles gives your lower body more power to maintain balance while executing their walking abilities. This benefit is exactly what performing calf raises can deliver to your body. They also help in pumping a great volume of blood up from your legs to your upper body and brain, so that you no longer deal with fainting or getting light-headed when standing still for long

- Other targeted areas: Toes, ankle.
- Length of workout: 5 mins
- Time duration for resting periods: 10 -20 secs in-between each set.
- Estimated calorie burn: 23 calories

Instructions

- Begin by standing upright with your feet slightly apart and your hands lightly holding onto a chair for balance and support.
- Pressing your toes, raise up on your toes as high as you comfortably can.
- Take a deep breath in and draw in your abdominals as you lift yourself.
- Hold that position for 2 -5 seconds and then return to the starting position.
- complete 4 sets of 5 reps.

Level up: To increase the difficulty of this exercise, let go of the chair, and if that is too hard for you, use a finger or one hand to hold on with. Doing this will even help improve your balance at a faster rate.

Precautions

- Make sure your body remains still as you raise yourself up.
- If you have balance problems, keep your feet apart
- Don't forget to inhale during the upward movement phase and exhale during the downward movement phase.

Bent-Over Row

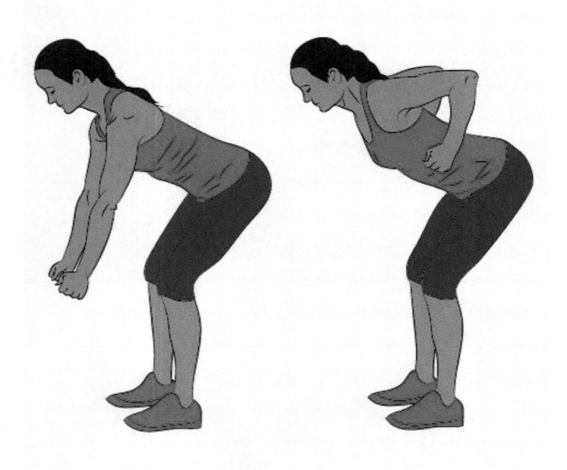

60. Bent-Over Row

Bent over rows are full-body strength-training exercises that help you to improve your ability to lift and pull. By doing so, it becomes easier for you to lift a bag of sugar, empty the trash, or open up a stubborn door. These exercises basically target and strengthen your upper arm and shoulders while increasing the range of motions in those areas.

- Other targeted areas: Back and Core
- Length of workout: 6 mins
- Time duration for resting periods: 20 - 30 secs in-between each set
- Estimated calorie burn: 46 calories

Instructions

- Start by standing up tall next to a firm chair with one hand placed on it.
- Now take a step back from the chair, while slightly bending your knees, and hinging at the hips.
- Still maintaining that position, bend forward with your back straight and one arm straight by your side.
- Now bending at the elbow, pull that arm up behind your back.
- Hold for 1-3 seconds and then return to the start position.
- Repeat 5 times with that arm and then alternate arms. Go for 2-3 sets of 5 reps on each arm.

Level up: Fill up your empty hands with dumbbells that are fit for your strength level.

Precautions

- As you lift your arm up, make sure to squeeze your shoulder blades.
- Focus on getting the form right before going on to complete the reps.

PART TWO:

STABILITY AND BALANCE

61. Tai Chi 8-form

Originated in China a long time ago, Tai Chi is a gentle, slow, and flowing form of exercise that provides real and substantial benefits for both your body and mind as seniors.

This gentle form of exercise is excellent for improving your body flexibility, balance coordination, and strength. By doing these, loosens your tight joints and helps alleviate arthritis pains. If you're a stroke and heart attack survivor, the tai chi movement is a sure way to recover at a faster rate.

Practicing the Tai Chi 8 Forms Movement gives you the essential foundational knowledge that you need to progress to the more advanced Tai Chi 24 Forms movement in terms of proper breathing, posture, balance, and concentration.

- Length of workout: 4 mins
- Estimated calorie burn: 68 calories.

Instructions

1. Commencement Pose

- Stand still with your hands by your side and your two feet together.
- Slowly lift your left foot and step sideways to the left. Make sure to lift your heel first before your toes but land on toes first.
- Move your arms to shoulder level with your palms facing down.
- While slightly bending your elbows, press your palms downwards to your abdominal level. At the same time, bend your knee slightly.

Reverse Reeling Forearms

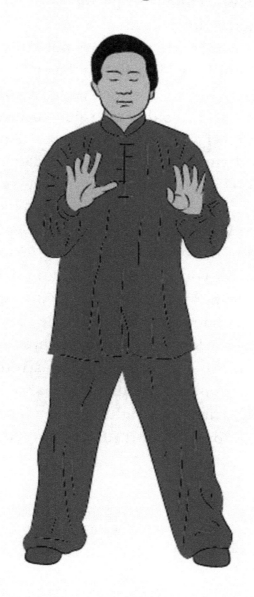

2. Reverse reeling forearms

- From the commencement pose, turn your body to the right corner while, dropping your palms with your fingers facing downwards.
- Now note that both arms are not fully extended. Your elbows should also be slightly bent.
- Slightly turn your chest to the right corner, stretch out both palms to the side and raise your arms upwards to shoulder level with your right hand at the rear right corner and your left hand at 12 O'clock.
- Bend your right elbow to raise your right hand, simultaneously turning your neck to look at 12 O'clock.
- Next, turn your body back to 12 O'clock and push your right hands with your palm facing forward in this same direction. As you do this, pull your left hand lower to the waist level with your palm facing upwards.
- Turn your body to the left side at the same time, dropping your left hands with fingers facing downwards.
- Turning your neck to the left side, stretch your left hand out to the side and lift it to your shoulder level. At the same time, turn your right palm to face upwards.
- Repeat the fourth and fifth steps on your left side.

Brush Knee Push

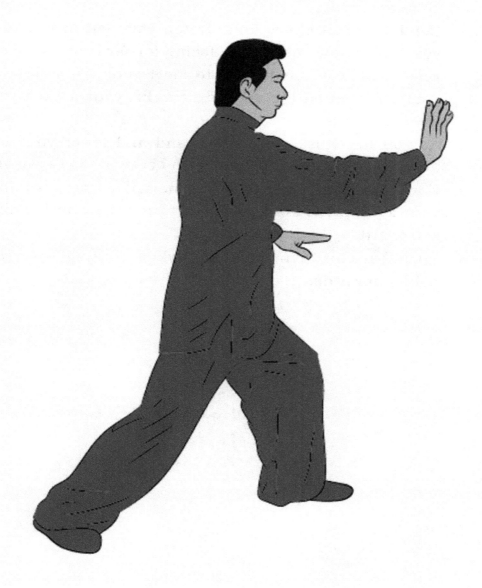

3. Brush knee push

- Still standing on your slightly bent knees, stretch out your right hand with your palm facing upwards to your shoulder level.

- Bend your left elbow and stretch your left arm across your chest with your palm facing forward. At the same time, pull your left heel in to meet your right. Raising your left heel off the ground first, lift your leg towards the side.

- As you lift, raise your right hand and lower your left arm. So, you expand the space in between the two arms.

- Now turn your body towards the left corner, bending your left knee to 90 degrees with your right heel sliding backward.

- Push back on your right leg while turning your left palms upwards.

Part the Wild Horse's Mane

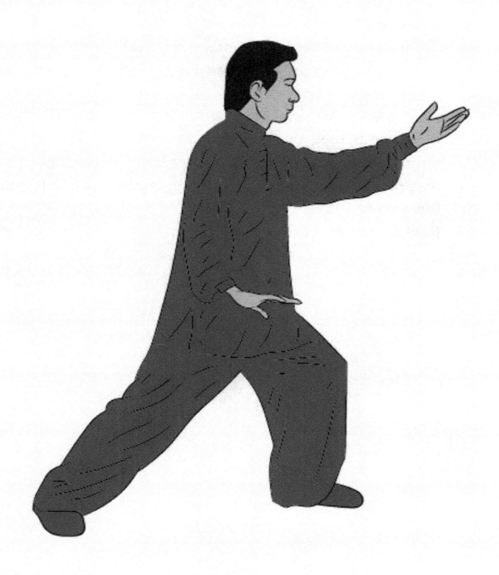

4. Part the wild horse's mane

- Stand upright with your body facing the left corner.
- Raise your right hand to the top with your palm facing down and your left hand on the bottom with your palm facing up.
- Sit on your left knee and step your right leg towards 12 O'clock; bring your left hand lower and raise your right hand up.
- Shift backward and press your left heel into the floor, lifting your toes.
- Maintaining that pose, turn your body to the right.
- Stepping in with your left leg bringing your left hand forward too.
- Now repeat on your left side.

Wave Hands Like Clouds

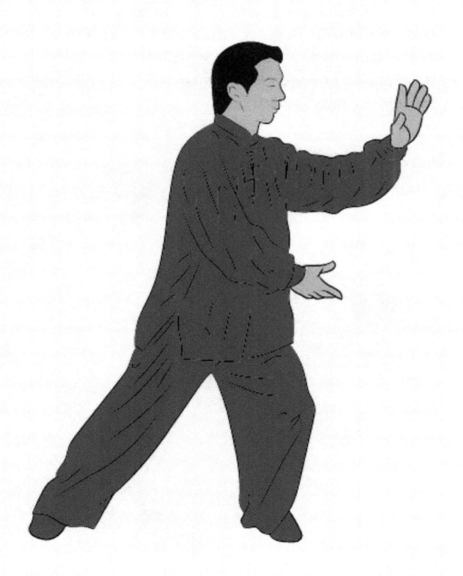

5. Wave hands like clouds

- Stand with your right hand on top and your left hand at the bottom, bending both elbows.
- Extend your right leg to the side and then shift your body weight on that leg, then step in with your left leg at the same time switching your hands.
- Now shift your weight to your left leg and repeat the movement on your left side.

Rooster Stands on One Leg

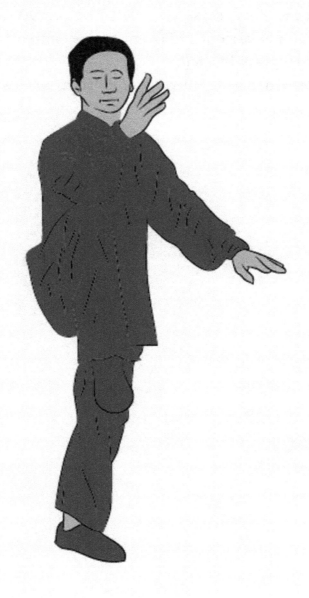

6. Rooster stands on one leg

- Stand upright with your arms by your side.
- Bending your elbow, extending your left arm up. At the same time, raise your left knee to 90 degrees.
- Then lower both of them at the same time, stepping back with your left leg.
- Repeat the same with your right arm and leg.

Kick with Heel

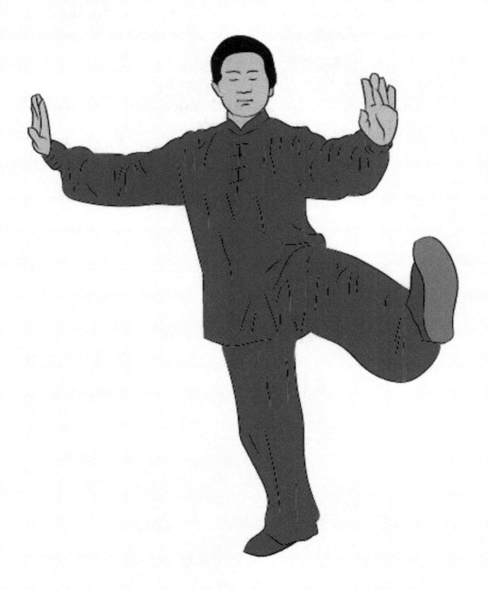

7. Kick with Heel

- Standing with your left leg in front and your right leg a step backward, extend your hands forward
- Then move back slightly and then lift your knee to 90 degrees crossing your hands across each other.
- Then expand your hands and kick your raised foot forward, lowering them to the ground.
- Switch to your other leg and repeat the movement.

Grasp the Peacock's Tail

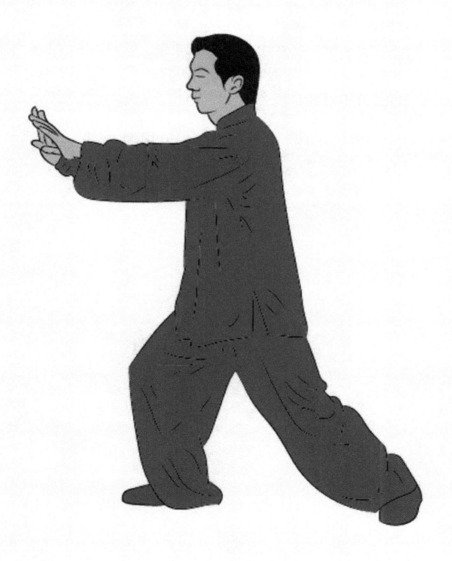

8. Grasp the peacock's Tail

- Begin with your right hand on top and your left hand on the bottom.
- Then lift your right leg to the side with your right knee slightly bent forward.
- Now turn your body to the side, shifting your weight forward and extending your two hands to grasp the imaginary peacock's tail, and pulling it back to the other side.
- Then release and gently free the bird with a push.

Cross Hands

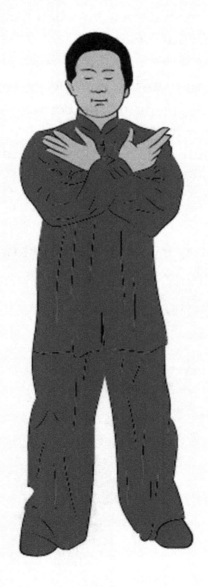

9. Cross Hands

- Stand and step your right leg to the side.
- Place both hands above your hands with palms facing outwards; the distance between your hands should be the width of your head.
- Slowly relax your shoulders and elbows as you lower your hands to drawing a circle as you go.
- Bring your right leg to the center to make it shoulder-length apart with your left leg.
- Bring both hands in your front of your shoulder's palms facing downwards and cross them.

Precautions

- Make sure that every movement is slow and controlled.

62. Tai Chi 24-form

Now that we have understood the basics, here are the more advanced but simplified 24 Tai Chi forms. They offer the same benefits as the other 8 postures we previously discussed but in a broader range

- Length of workout: 6 minutes
- Estimated calorie burn:

Instructions

Section 1

Opening stance / Qi Shi

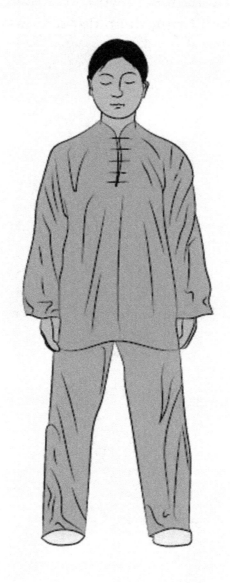

1. Commencing Form/Qishi

- Stand upright, feet together.
- Move you left leg sideways for balance.
- Raise both hands to your shoulder level, evenly and slowly. Then bring them down slowly.

Part the horse mane (left & right) / Ye Ma Fen Zong

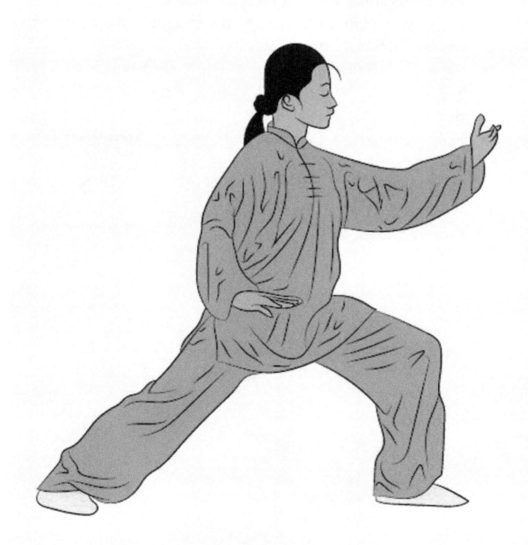

2. Part the horse mane (left & right) / Ye Ma Fen Zong

- Continuously move your weight to the right leg to form an empty step and hold a ball, take a bow.
- Raise your left hand to shoulder level and right-hand presses down to hip area.
- Rotate the left foot, form the empty step and hold a ball.
- Take a bow. Right hand goes up and left hand goes down.
- Rotate the right foot. Form an empty step and hold a ball.
- Take a bow step, left hand goes up and right hand goes done.

White crane spreads it's wings / Bai He Liang Chi

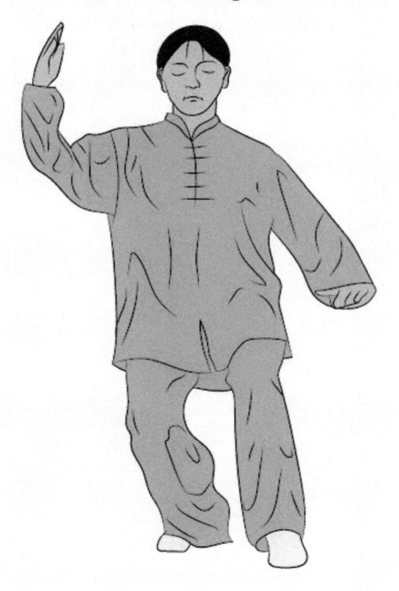

3. White crane spreads its wings / Bai He Liang Chi

- Right foot takes a step. Form an empty step and hold a ball, the right hand goes up and the left hand goes down.

Brush knee, twist steps / Lou Xi Ao Bu

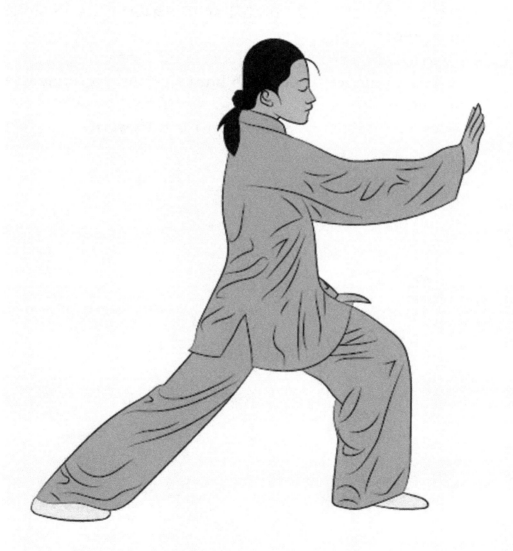

4. Brush knee, twist steps / Lou Xi Ao Bu

- Rotate the right knee. Both hands perform a semicircle movement.
- Brush left knee and push right hand forward.
- Rotate the left knee. Both hands perform a semicircle movement.
- Brush right knee and push left hand forward.
- Rotate to the left knee. Both hands perform a semicircle movement.
- Brush left knee and push right hand forward.

Strum the lute / Shou Hui Pi Ba

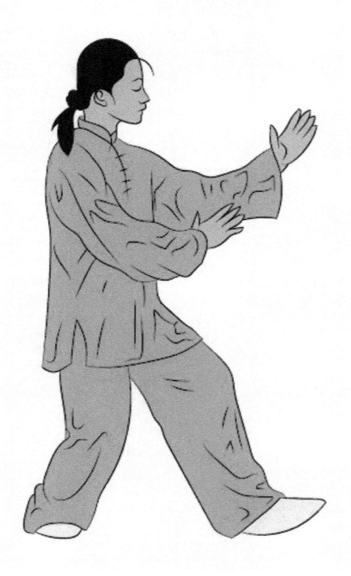

5. Strum the lute / Shou Hui Pi Ba

- Right foot takes a step, raise hands and lean on the heel.

Repulse the monkey (left & right) / Dao Zhuang Gong

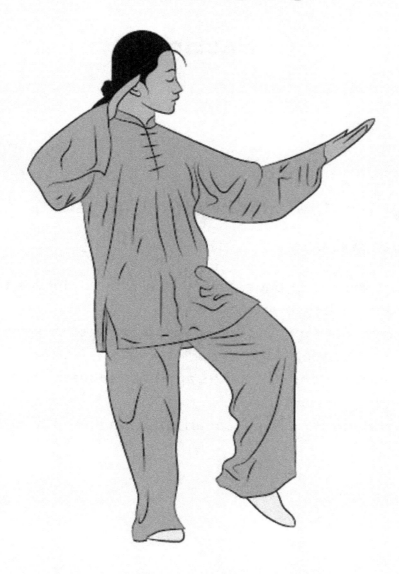

Section 2

6. Repulse the monkey (left & right) / Dao Zhuang Gong

- Left foot, step back, right hand rotates, moves up and then pushes forward.
- Right foot steps back, left hand rotates, moves up and then push forward.
- Step back and roll hands again. Take a step back again and roll hands.
- Rotate to the foot. Form an empty step and hold a ball.

Grasp the peacock's tail (left) / Zuo Lan Que Wei

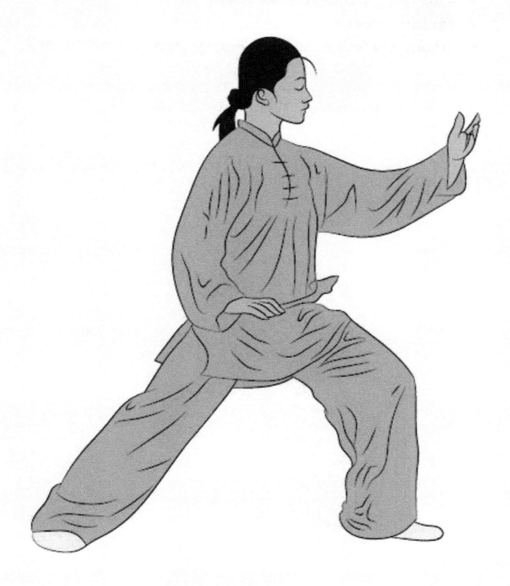

7. Grasp the peacock's tail (left) / Zuo Lan Que Wei

- Take a bow-like step. Deflect. Push.
- Pull in. Press.
- Rotate the left heel form, empty step and hold a ball.

Grasp the peacock's tail (right) / You Lan Que Wei

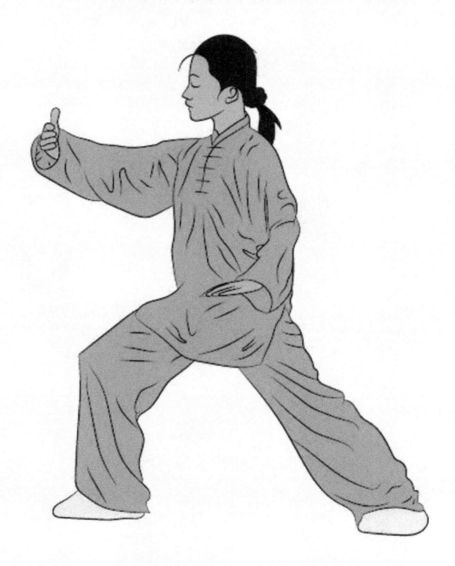

8. Grasp the peacock's tail (right) / You Lan Que Wei

- Take a bold step and ward off. Deflect. Push. Pull in. Press.

Single whip / Dan Bian

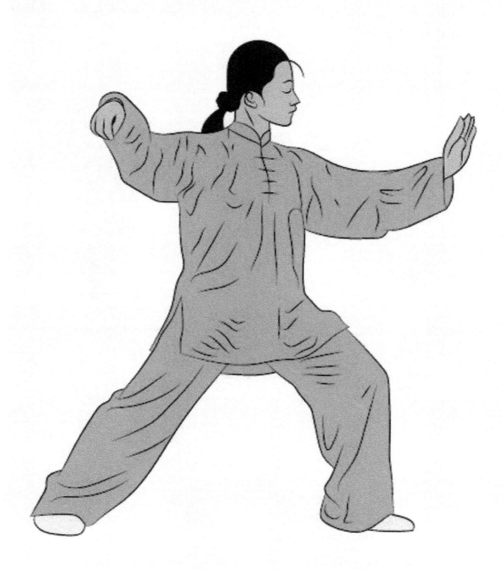

9. Single whip / Dan Bian

- Rotate both arms. Right hand bunches a hook, then forms an empty step.
- Take a left step, rotate and push left hand lean on left foot and grind right foot.

Waving hands like clouds / Yun Shou

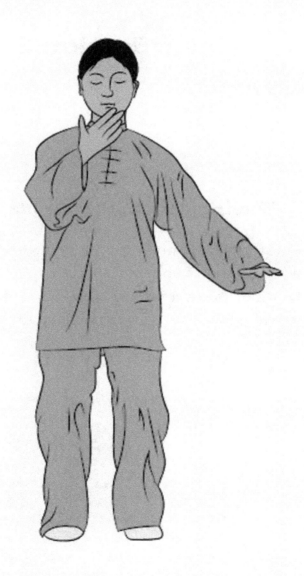

Section 3

10. Waving hands like clouds / Yun Shou

- Rotate the left heel, move the right foot to the left and wave hands to the left.
- Left foot takes a lateral step. Wave hands to the right.
- Wave hands like clouds twice again.

Single whip / Dan Bian

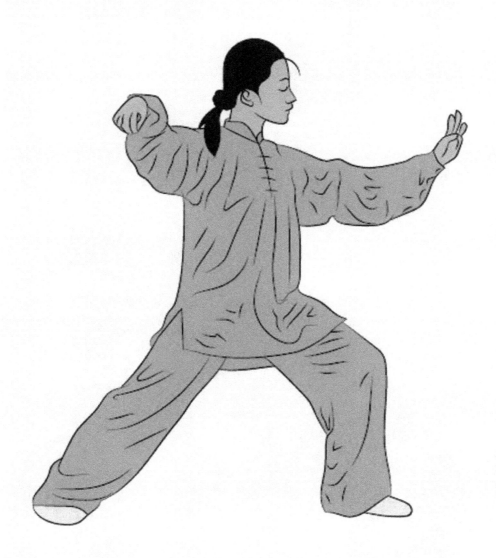

11. Single whip / Dan Bian

- Bunch a hook and form an empty step.
- Take a left step, rotate and push left hand and lean left foot and grind right foot.

High pat the horse / Gao Tan Ma

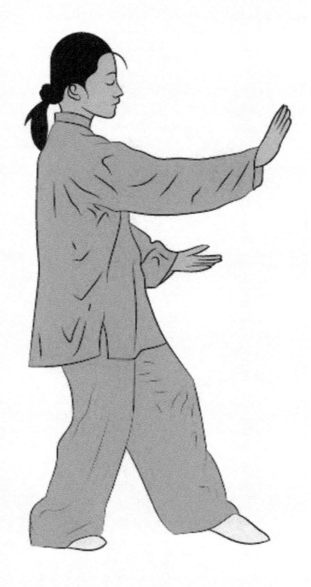

12. High pat the horse / Gao Tan Ma

- Right foot takes a step and forms an empty step.
- Right palm moves forward.
- Take a left bow step and then form an empty step.

Right heel kick / You Deng Jiao

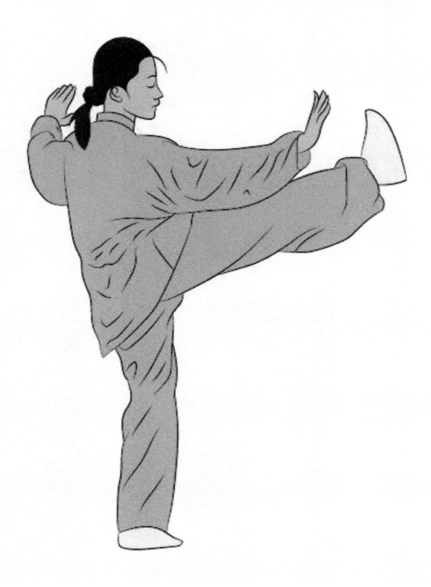

13. Right heel kick / You Deng Jiao

- Cross hands in front of the chest, raise the right knee and then kick with right heel.
- Palm separate and move outward.

Double punch to the Ears / Shuang Feng Guan Er

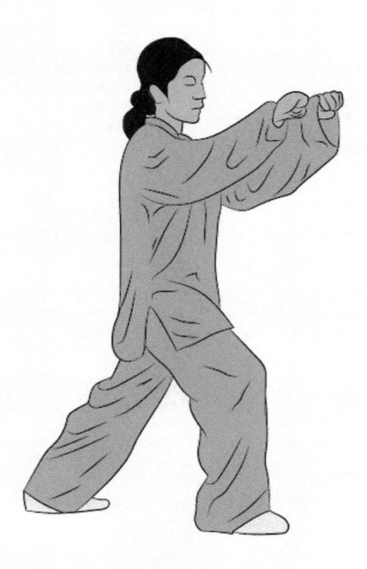

14.Double Punch to the Ears / Shuang Feng Guan

- Drop the right foot; draw both palms back
- Take a bold step, and change your palm into fists and strike on the opponent.

Turn round and left heel kick / Zhuang Shen Zuo Deng Jiao

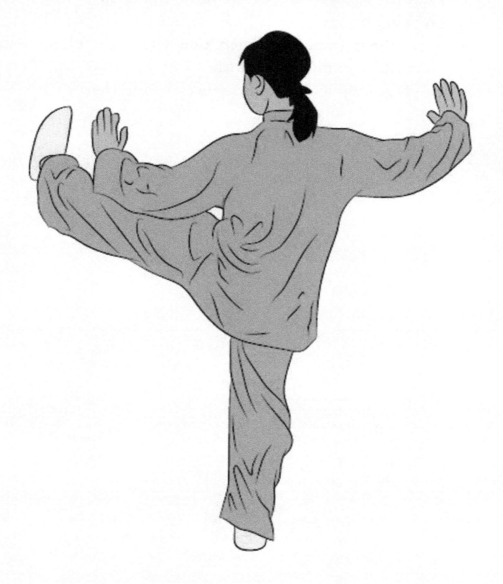

15. Turn round and left heel kick / Zhuang Shen Zuo Deng Jiao

- Rotate the right heel and form the empty step while crossing hands.
- Raise the left knee and then kick with the left heel. Palm separate and move outward.
- Left leg pulls in, left hand moves to the right axilla.

Creep down and golden cock stand on one leg (left) / Zuo Xia Shi Du Li

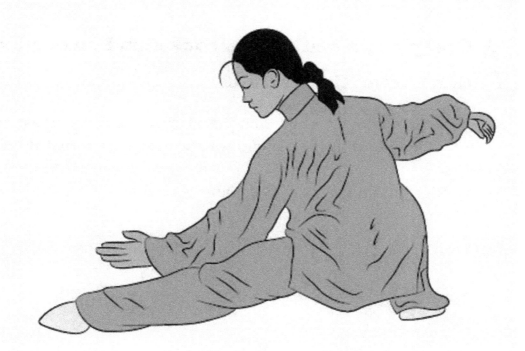

Section 4

16. Creep down and golden cock stand on one leg (left) / Zuo Xia Shi Du Li

- Take a crouch step. Left hand threads from chest to abdomen along the inside of the leg; stand on the left leg.
- Right hand goes up. Left hand goes down.

Creep down and golden cock stand on one leg (right) / You Xia Shi Du Li

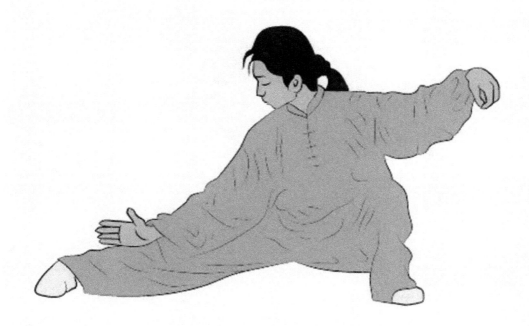

17. Creep down and golden cock stand on one leg (right) / You Xia Shi Du Li

- Land on the right toe. Rotate the left heel, right hand moves to the left axilla.
- Right leg takes a crouch step. Right palm front chest to abdomen along the inside of the leg.
- Stand on the right leg, left hand goes up, right hand goes down.
- Take a left step. Form empty step and hold a ball.

Fair lady works the shuttle (left & right) / Zuo You Yu Nv Chuan Shuo

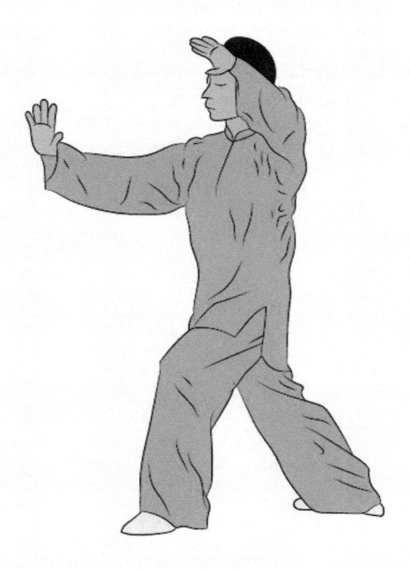

18. Fair lady works the shuttle (left & right) / Zuo You Yu Nv Chuan Shuo

- Right foot takes a bold step, right arm and rotates and blocks up, left palm pushes out.
- Rotate the right, heel form an empty step and hold a ball.
- Left foot takes a step, left arm rotates and blocks up right palm pushes out.
- Right foot takes a half step raise both hands

Needle at the bottom of the sea /
Hai Di Zhen

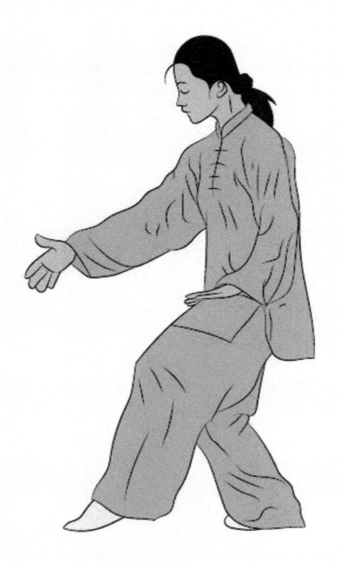

19. Needle at the bottom of the sea / Hai Di Zhen

- Brush the left knee and needle the left hand down.

Fan through back / Shan Tong Bi

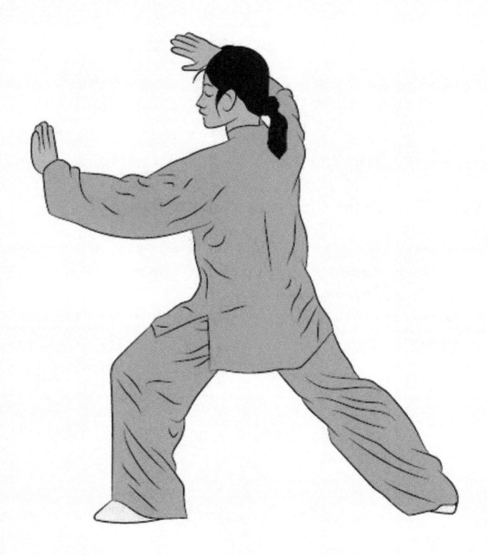

Section 5

20. Fan through back / Shan Tong Bi

- Raise hand and left foot takes a bow.
- Right hand brought up and left palm pushed forward. x Rotate the left heel.
- Then right fist moves out and the foot takes a step forward.

Turn round block, parry and punch / Zhuang Shen Ban Lan Chui

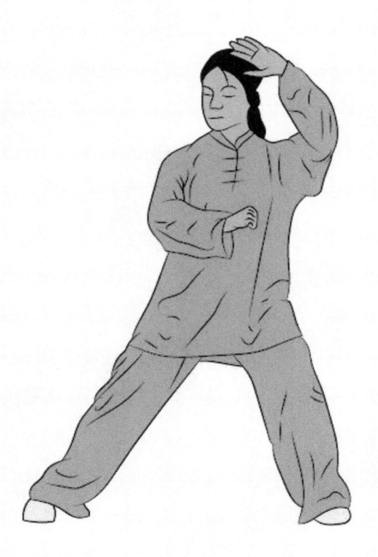

21. Turn round block, parry and punch / Zhuang Shen Ban Lan Chui

- Left foot takes a step forward with the left-hand doing a perry and then the right fist forward.

Apparent close up / Ru Feng Si Bi

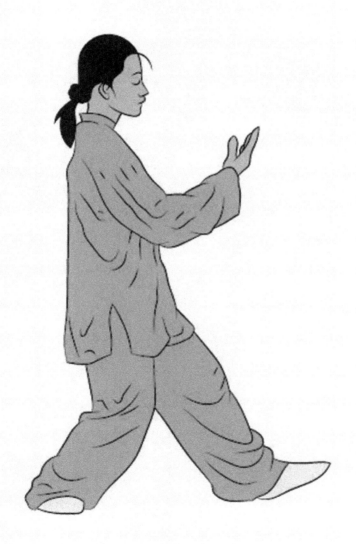

22. Apparent close up / Ru Feng Si Bi

- Both hands pull inward and downward.
- Then press both hands upward and forward.

Cross hand / Shi Zi Shou

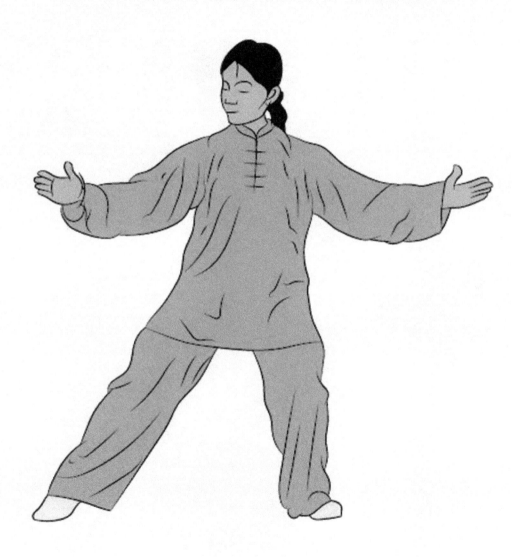

23. Cross hand / Shi Zi Shou

- Rotate the left heel and then rotate the right.
- Open the arms and separate the hands.
- Cross the hands in front of the chest.

Close stance / Shou Shib

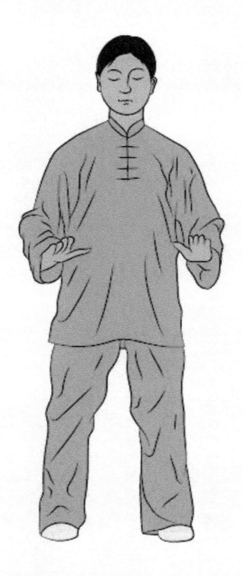

24. Close stance / Shou Shi

- Press both hands down gently until they rest beside the hips.
- Slowly put feet together. And gently put hands along the sides.

Level up: You can always up to the 88 forms. Although it was condensed to the 24 forms, doing the 88 forms offers improved benefits.

Precautions

- The exercise includes a lot of rotations, be wary of this to avoid slips. Ty to perform the Tai Chi 24 forms on a not so smooth surface with flat shoes on.

Step-Ups

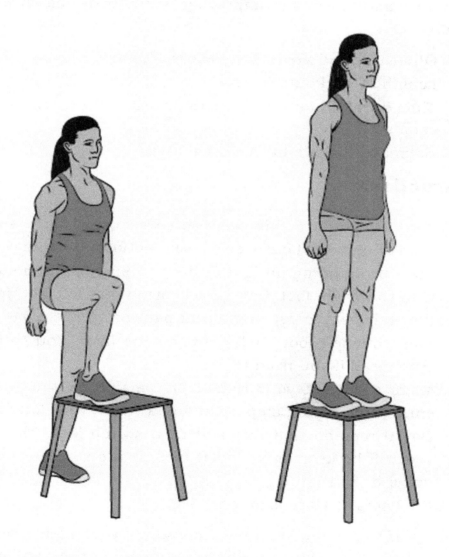

63. Step Ups

For most seniors, step-ups are the perfect exercise that comes to mind for strengthening your legs using the stairs in your home. By strengthening the muscles that support the knee, you are simultaneously improving your body balance and stability.

- Other targeted areas: hip flexors, thighs.
- Length of workout: 7 mins
- Time duration for resting periods: 30 - 40 secs in-between each set.
- Estimated calorie burn: 51 calories

Instructions

- You can perform this exercise either on a staircase with rails or on a workout step/raised platform if you have one.
- Start by standing upright at the bottom step, then step up with your right foot. Now, slowly bring your left foot up onto the stair next to your right and pause a bit.
- Step your left foot back down on the floor. You can hold onto a rail if you need to.
- Make sure that your right foot remains on the step the entire time as you step up and down with your left foot.
- Do 10 reps on that foot and then switch legs. This time, you will be keeping your left foot on the step as you step up with the right leg.
- Do 3 sets of 10 reps on each leg.

Level up: If you're holding onto the rails of your staircase, then try letting go of it to make the exercise more intense and improve your balance at the same time.

Precautions

- If you're struggling with severe knee problems or this exercise is too painful, it is highly recommended that you skip it.

Ball Tap

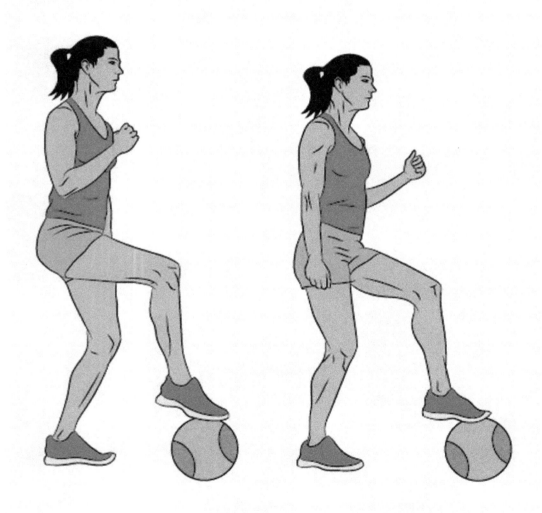

64. Ball Tap

Ball tap is another effective move that is great for the core as well as for balance and stability. Basically, it involves the use of any kind of small ball. If you don't have a ball, you can improvise by using a large book.

- Other targeted areas: Back, core
- Length of workout: 7 mins
- Time duration for resting periods: 20 - 30 secs in-between each set.
- Estimated calorie burn: 23 calories

Instructions

- Sit up in a sturdy chair with your back straight. Try not to rest against the back of the chair.
- Place a ball in front of both feet.
- Keeping your abs tight, slowly lift your right foot and tap the top of the ball.
- Lower it back down to the floor. That's one rep.
- Go for 10 reps before switching sides and doing the same with your left foot.

Level up: Consider placing your hands behind your head, as you perform this exercise.

Precautions

- Though the exercise seems quite easy, you need to keep your movements slow and steady.

The Basic Bridge

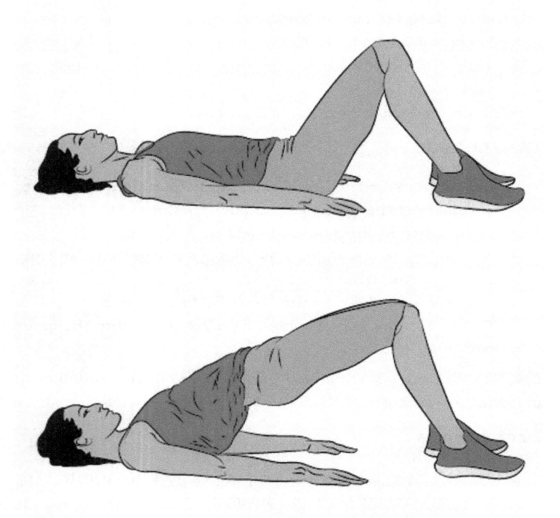

65. The Basic Bridge

The basic bridge is an effective strength-training and stability exercise that is best described as simplicity in itself. The basic bridge targets and isolates your abdominal muscles and the muscles of the lower back and hip. This, in turn, helps in improving your core and spinal stabilization.

- Other targeted areas: gluteus (butt) muscles, abs, and hamstrings
- Length of workout: 6 mins
- Time duration for resting periods: 20 - 30 secs
- Estimated calorie burn: 27 calories

Instructions

- Begin by lying down on your back with your hands at your sides, knees bent, and feet flat on the floor under your knees.
- Before you push up, tighten your abdominal and butt muscles by pushing your low back into the ground.
- Maintaining that pose, raise your hips up while squeezing your core and pulling your belly button back toward your spine. Your body should form a straight line from your knees to shoulders.
- Hold that position for 10-20 seconds, and then return to your starting position.
- Complete 2-3 sets of 5 reps, taking rest where necessary.

Level up: To increase the difficulty of this movement, you can add an exercise band, dumbbell, or exercise ball into the workout routine.

Precautions

- Avoid raising your hips too high as that can make you extend your lower back too much.
- It's okay if you can't hold the pose for up to 30 seconds. Always keep in mind that it is better to hold the correct position for a shorter time frame than to stay in an incorrect position for a longer time.

PART THREE:

BALANCE AND COORDINATION

66. Qigong Knee Rotation Exercise

Adopted from an ancient Chinese practice, Qigong exercises are gentle low-impact exercises that are highly recommended for seniors. This particular Qigong exercise targets your knee. It not only does help to improve balance and reduce falls but also fits well into any training routine. Besides its physical benefits, this exercise promotes reduced stress, clearer thinking, and a stronger immune system.

- Other targeted areas: Hamstrings, back
- Length of workout: 4 mins
- Time duration for resting periods: 5 - 10 secs in-between each set.
- Estimated calorie burn: 23 calories

Instructions

- Stand up nice and tall with your back and shoulder relaxed; your feet shoulder-width apart.
- Bend your knees and place your hands on the knee caps
- Gently and slowly begin rotating your knees inwards 6 times then rotate outwards 6 times.
- Complete 2 sets of 12 reps.

Precautions

- Make sure your weight is evenly distributed on your legs before you start this exercise.
- If you cannot do this movement while standing, it is okay to sit.

Quadruped Opposite Arm and Leg Balance

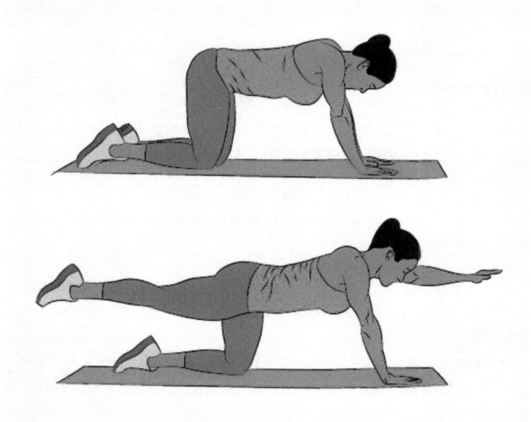

67. Quadruped Opposite Arm and Leg Balance

This exercise is another strength-training movement for seniors that improves balance and coordination in the body, most especially in your back and abdominals.

- Other targeted areas: Glutes, hamstrings, shoulders
- Length of workout: 5 mins
- Time duration for resting periods: 20 - 30 secs in-between each set.
- Estimated calorie burn: 40 calories

Instructions

- Get on all fours with your hands directly underneath your shoulders and knees under your hips.
- While keeping your back flat and drawing in your abdominals, lift your left hand to reach straight in front of your shoulder while lifting your right foot straight behind your hip.
- Now, hold for 2 - 5 seconds, and then lower your hand and foot toward the floor to return to start.
- Repeat on the opposite side with your right hand and left foot.
- Complete 3 sets of 7 reps on both sides of your body.

Level up: Use an elastic band to add more resistance around your thigh areas

Precautions

- As you extend your leg back, do not over arch your back at the top of the movement.

- A great way to do that is to squeeze your glutes for more stability.
- Also, ensure that your hips do not shift side to side during the exercise.

Balance on One Leg

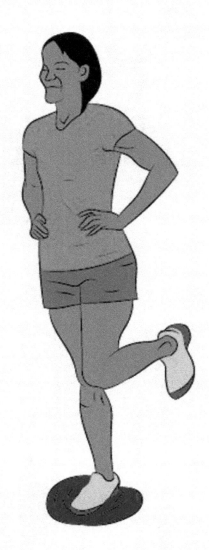

68. Rock the Boat/Balance on One Leg

As an elderly person and a daily walker, Rock the boat exercise will be quite a simple one for you. It basically focuses on improving your standing balance and coordination.

- Other targeted areas: Knee, hip flexors
- Length of workout: 6 mins
- Time duration for resting periods: 20 - 30 secs in-between each set.
- Estimated calorie burn: 32 calories

Instructions

- Stand upright with your feet hip-width apart.
- Ensure that both feet are pressed into the ground firmly, transfer your weight to your right foot and slowly lift your left leg off the ground.
- Hold that position for 5 - 30 seconds. Then slowly put your foot back onto the ground, then transfer your weight to that foot.
- With the same level of control, lift your opposite leg.
- Start by completing 2-3 sets of 8 reps per side, then work your way up to doing more repetitions.

Level up: As you work up your balance game, you can add a set of dumbbells to make it more fun but still challenging.

Precautions

- Make sure to wear your walking shoes, and stand on a yoga mat to give your feet a little extra cushion.
- If you are having a problem with balancing, you can use a chair for support.

Leg Swings

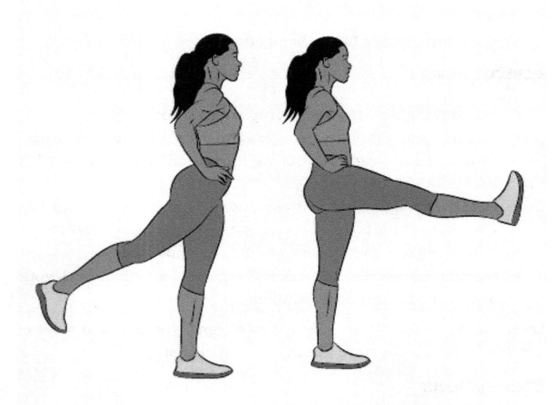

69. Leg Swings

Leg swings are another great balance and strength-training exercise that is quite effective for seniors. This exercise challenges your balance by disrupting your ability to keep your torso over your ankle.

- Other targeted areas: Hamstrings, glutes
- Length of workout: 6 mins
- Time duration for resting periods: 20 - 30 secs in between each set.
- Estimated calorie burn: 28 calories

Instructions

- Begin by starting upright with a chair at your side for safety.
- Now, press your left leg firmly on the floor and use it for balance as you swing your outside leg forward and backward in a smooth motion.
- As you swing, keep holding onto the chair with your ribs lifted and your head forward. x Swing for one minute on each side before taking a break and going for 2 more rounds.

Level up: When you have worked up your balance abilities to an extent, let go of the chair and perform these movements independently.

Precautions

- Try to have a family member or personal trainer present to assist when doing these balance exercises.
- Focus on maintaining your center of gravity over your planted foot.

Around the Clock

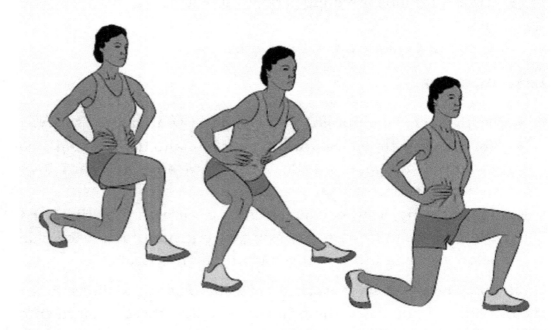

70. Around the Clock

This exercise aims to improve your static or standing balance. It helps increase the strength in your ankles and hips joints, which are vital in keeping your body stable. It also gives you the chance to expand the range of motion of your upper body. Just like the previous exercises, all you need here is to get into comfortable loose-fitting clothing and a pair of smooth bottom shoes!

- Other targeted areas: Shoulder and back.
- Length of workout: 6 mins
- Time duration for resting periods: 10 -20 secs in-between each set.
- Estimated calorie burn: 30 calories

Instructions

- Begin by standing up and holding on to a chair with your left hand.
- Envision a clock by your side with 12 in front of you and 6 behind.
- Now shift your weight onto your left leg and lift your right leg as you stretch out your right arm to the side, hitting 12 o'clock.
- Next, rotate your hands like a clock as you try to reach 3 and 6 o'clock.
- Repeat with the other side. Complete 2 sets of 6 reps on both sides.

Level up: Start by simply holding on with one finger or even let go of the chair completely. You can also add a one-pound weight to your wrist or ankle for a more challenging workout.

Precautions

- Avoid reaching too far especially if you have shoulder pain. If you cannot reach 6 o'clock, or if it is painful, stop at 3 o'clock.
- Remember to breathe normally while exercising, in through the nose and out through the mouth.

One Legged Squat

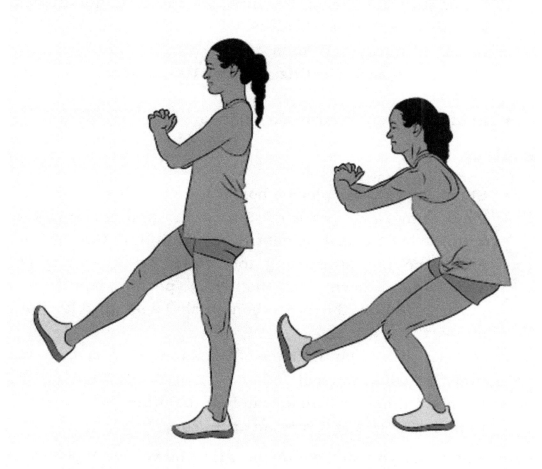

71. One-Legged Squat

As a senior, adding one-legged squats to your strength-training program is a great way to simultaneously develop strength, balance, coordination, and core stability. It also helps to tone and strengthen your legs and core muscles.

- Other targeted areas: the hips, hamstrings, quadriceps, gluteus maximus, and calves.
- Length of workout: 5 mins
- Time duration for resting periods: 10 -20 secs in-between each set.
- Estimated calorie burn: 38 calories

Instructions

- Stand upright and place a box or low chair behind you.
- Plant your right foot firmly on the ground beneath you, with the left leg slightly bent or straight out in front of you.
- Raise the non-supporting foot from the floor slightly. Slowly sink down into the squat position until your buttocks touch the box, then push back up with your supporting leg.
- Make sure to keep the knee of the supporting leg centered over the ball of the foot
- Repeat 5 times and then switch to the other leg.
- Complete 2 sets of 5 reps on each leg.

Level up: Once you are confident that you've developed your coordination, and balance enough to make this exercise more intense, switch to holding a dumbbell or kettlebell in your hands while doing it.

Precautions

- As you squat, your knee should not extend beyond your toes.
- This exercise demands that every one of your moves is slow.
- To make sure that you get the correct form, perform this exercise in front of a mirror.

Single Leg Dead Lift

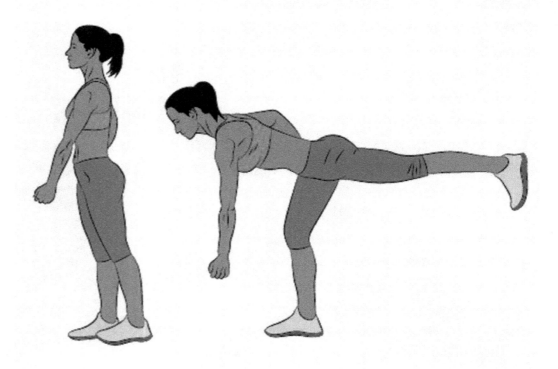

72. Single-Leg Deadlift

Performing single-leg deadlift consistently and correctly simply equals greater balance, flexibility, and stability for you even in the face of aging factors.

- Other targeted areas: Hamstrings, gluteus maximus, gluteus medius, ankles, and the core.
- Length of workout: 8 mins
- Time duration for resting periods: 30 -49 secs in-between each set.
- Estimated calorie burn: 52 calories

Instructions

- Start by standing with your right leg firmly planted on the ground beneath you and the left leg bent up behind you.
- Start hinging at your waist as you slowly bend over as you lift and stretch your left leg out behind you.
- Your right knee should be slightly bent with your arms straight. Your body should also be in a straight line from the top of your head to the bottom of your left foot
- Stop bending and pause when your torso is almost parallel to the floor.
- Slowly, rise back up and then repeat 2-3 sets of 5 reps on each leg, resting when necessary.

Level up. Add dumbbells or kettlebells to the opposite arm of the leg on the ground.

Precautions

- Keep your back neutral and avoid rounding your spine as you bend. Imagine that you have a glass of water resting on your low back when your torso becomes parallel to the floor so you must ensure that the water doesn't spill.

Baz Thompson

Stretches - Flexibility & Relaxation

To attain overall functional independence as you age, you cannot only focus on strength training. Thus, just like we have discussed strength-training exercises that are great at improving balance, stability, and coordination, we will now focus on strength-training exercises that promote the mobility and flexibility of your muscles, tendons, and the connective tissue surrounding your muscles and joints.

Chest and Arm Stretch

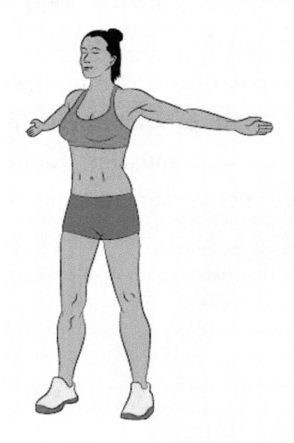

73. Chest and Arm Stretch

Poor posture while sitting or standing is quite common with elderly persons and even young ones too. Thus, it often leads to stiffness and tensions in the muscles of the chest becoming tight. The chest and arm exercise help to properly stretch and lengthen those tight muscles. Eventually, your posture will also improve.

- Other targeted areas: Shoulder, back.
- Length of workout: 4 mins
- Time duration for resting periods: 5 -10 secs in-between each set
- Estimated calorie burn: 15 calories.

Instructions

- Start by getting seated and extending both arms to the side, palms facing forward. Inhale as you do this.
- Now, slowly reach back with your hands until you feel a stretch across your chest and front of your arms.
- Pause briefly and slowly return to the starting position. Switch to the other side. Complete 3 sets of 5 reps.

Level up: Try performing these movements while standing up.

Precautions

- Use a wall if you are finding it difficult to hold your arms up without support. All you have to do is to put your hand on a wall and step forward until you feel a gentle stretch in your chest.
- Do not overstretch.

Hamstring/Calf Stretch

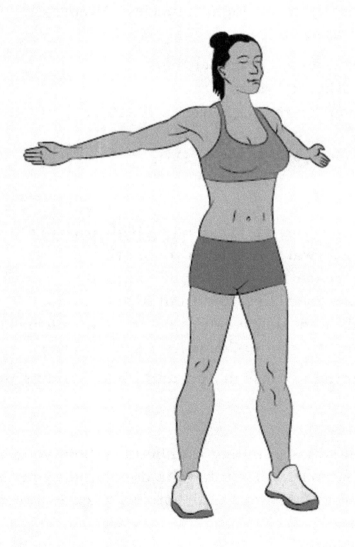

74. Hamstring/Calf Stretch

Remember that your hamstrings, which are the muscles on the back of your thigh. Thus, they are very important for your walking and standing abilities. Hamstring stretch helps relieve tension in your calves, which may cause your lower back pain and difficulty in walking.

- Other targeted areas: Upper and lower back.
- Length of workout: 4 mins
- Time duration for resting periods: 5 - 10 secs in-between each set
- Estimated calorie burn: 15 calories

Instructions

- Place your yoga mat on the floor and lie on your back.
- Extend your right leg perpendicular to your body.
- Keeping your left leg and hip stuck to the ground, grasp around the back of your thigh and slowly pull the leg towards you for 2 -5 seconds.
- Release and then lower your leg back to the ground. Repeat 5 times on your right leg before switching legs.
- Do 3 sets of 5 reps on each leg.

Level up: Try using a resistance band around your thighs.

Precautions

- Do not pull on your knee when stretching. x Remember to inhale and exhale as you stretch.

Quadriceps Stretch

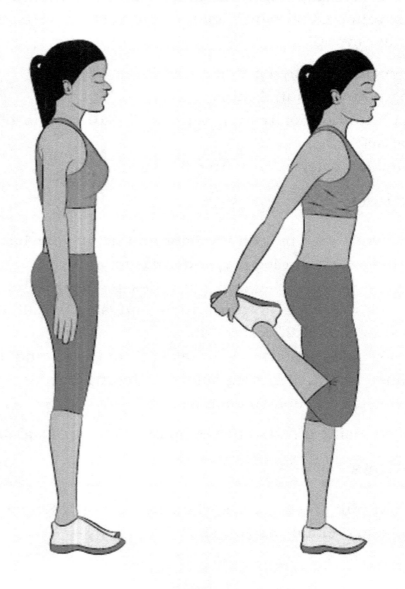

75. Quadriceps Stretch

This stretch works your quadriceps, which are large muscles on the front of the thigh. It increases your range of motion and flexibility in that area. This will ultimately improve your walking and standing stamina.

- Other targeted areas: Hamstrings, and back.
- Length of workout: 4 mins
- Time duration for resting periods: 5 - 10 secs in-between each set.
- Estimated calorie burn: 16 calories.

Instructions

- Start by lying on your side with your right knee bent and your foot behind you.
- With your hand, pull that foot towards your body until you feel a stretch.
- If you find it hard to reach your foot, you can use a belt or a towel to help.
- Repeat this 6 times before switching to your left leg.
- Completes 2-3 sets of 6 reps on each leg.

Level up: Perform these same motions in a standing position.

Precautions

- Draw in your abdominal muscles as you pull your foot.
- Pull to the point of tension and not to the point of pain.

Neck, Upper Back, And Shoulder Stretch

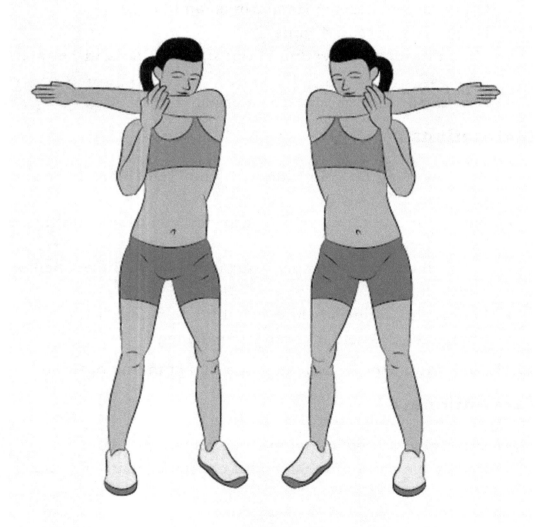

76. Neck, Upper Back and Shoulder Stretch

This exercise help improve flexibility and maintain mobility in your neck, shoulder and upper back simultaneously. By doing this, it also helps to improve your body posture and provide relief in your tight neck and shoulders.

- Other targeted areas: Core, arms.
- Length of workout: 5 mins
- Time duration for resting periods: 5 - 10 secs in-between each set.
- Estimated calorie burn: 19 calories

Instructions

- Start by standing in a comfortable standing position with your arms by your side.
- Cross your right arm straight across your chest to the opposite side.
- Then use your left arm to gently pull the outstretched right arm closer to your body.
- Hold for 5 - 10 secs and then repeat on the other side.
- Do 2-3 sets of 5 reps on both sides.

Precautions

- Never stretch your arm too much to the point of pain

Pec Stretches

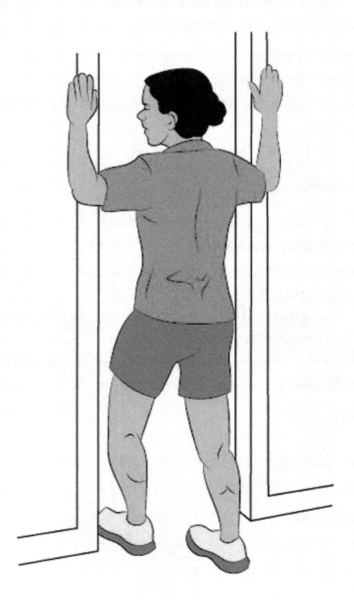

77. Standing Side Reach/Pec Stretches

This exercise offers you increased shoulder and trunk flexibility as well as a good balance. This will train your body to easily reach higher surfaces like the high shelf at home or the grocery store.

- Other targeted areas: Chest, core
- Length of workout: 4 mins
- Time duration for resting periods: 5 - 10 secs in-between each set.
- Estimated calorie burn: 15 calories.

Instructions

- Stand up and tall with your feet slightly wider than hip-width apart and knees slightly bent.
- As if you're reaching up to grab an object, reach your right hand up and out toward the same side while shifting weight to the leg of the same side,
- Maintain good balance as you reach out until you feel a stretch on the side of your trunk.
- Hold for 3 to 5 seconds, then return to the starting position and repeat it with the opposite arm.
- Do two sets of ten reps per side.

Level up: Try holding dumbbells of comfortable weights in your hands as you reach up and out.

Precautions

- Do not reach out your hands too far upwards as that will most likely put a strain on your lower back.
- Breathe normally in through your nose and out through your mouth.

Shoulder and Upper Back Stretch

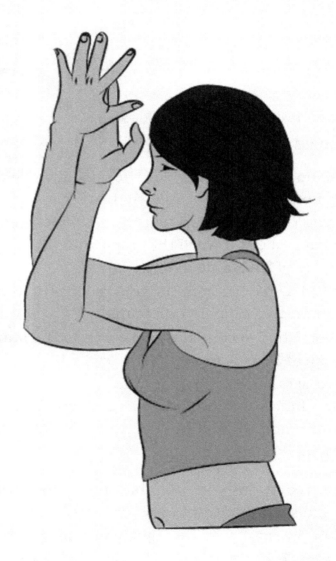

78. Shoulder and Upper Back Stretch

This movement basically focuses on increasing your shoulder and scapular range of motion. It also stretches your upper back and shoulder which in turn improves your reaching abilities.

- Other targeted areas: Chest
- Length of workout: 5 mins
- Time duration for resting periods: 10 - 20 secs in-between each set.
- Estimated calorie burn: 16 calories.

Instructions

- Sit up and comfortably in your chair.
- Then bring and bind your palms together in front of your chest, like you're about to pray.
- As you do this, take a deep breath in through your nose. Try to bring the air all the way down to your abdomen when breathing in.
- Now exhale as you bring your arms up with your palms still bound together. Straighten arms overhead with palms forward.
- Take a breath pause; then lower your arms out to the side and back to the starting position.
- Squeeze your shoulder blades as you bring your arms down.
- Complete 2-3 sets of 7 reps.

Level up: To make this exercise more intense, add one-pound wrist weights to your arms.

Precautions

- As you raise your hands, ensure that your forearms are kept together.
- Keep your chest raised and your movements slow.

Shoulder Rolls

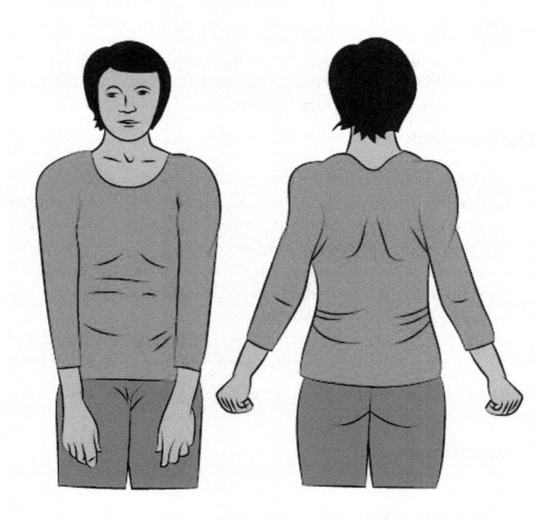

79. Shoulder Rolls

Rolling your shoulder helps find your end range motions in those joints and even expands your range of motion. By doing so, you can reduce the stiffness and tension, and at the same time improve the rate of flexibility in your shoulder joints.

- Other targeted areas: Upper back and Arms.
- Length of workout: 4 mins x Time duration for resting periods: 10 -20 secs in-between each set.
- Estimated calorie burn: 19 calories.

Instructions

- Get seated in a comfortable position on your chair.
- Keep your core tight, as you slowly but with control, raise your shoulders upwards, then backward, and finally downwards. That's one complete rep!
- Ensure you inhale and raise the ribs as you bring the shoulders up, then exhale as you lower it back to its normal position.
- Relax and then repeat 10 times. Before taking a break and going for 2 more sets of the same number of reps

Level up: Place dumbbells in your two hands while performing this exercise.

Precautions

- Depending on its severity, take a break or totally stop if you feel pain in your shoulder joints.
- Never hold your breath.

Neck Side Stretch

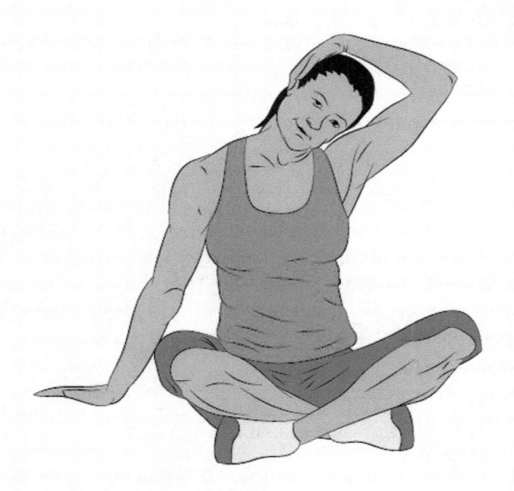

80. Neck Side Stretch

The neck side stretch helps relax the tension and stiffness in your neck by improving the range of motion in that area. This will in turn offer your relief for any neck pain.

- Other targeted areas: Upper back.
- Length of workout: 4 mins
- Time duration for resting periods: 5 - 10 secs in-between sets.
- Estimated calorie burn: 12 calories.

Instructions

- Get seated with your back straight against your chair.
- Bending your elbow, reach your right arm behind your back, and then place your left hand on top of your head.
- Now, gently tilt your head to the left. Hold for 5 seconds, then relax and repeat with the other side.
- Complete 3 sets of 5 reps on each set.

Level up: Focus on coordinating your breathing by exhaling during the stretch to relax your neck.

Precautions

- Do not hold the neck stretch for more than 5 seconds. If you have had a stroke in the past, then 2 to 3 seconds is enough.
- If you can't place your hand on top of your head, just simply but gently tilt it!
- Again, stretching should be relaxing so stop and take a break if you experience any pain.

Neck Rotation

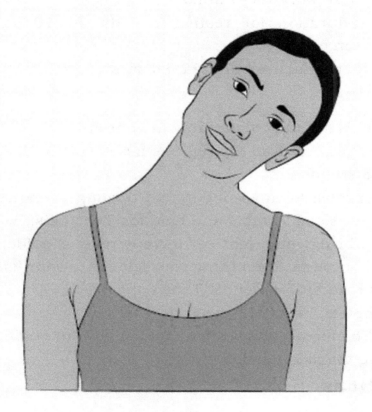

81. Neck Rotation

This exercise is an effective and safe way to relieve neck stiffness and pain, common problems of elderly people. It also helps in expanding the range of motions in your neck muscles and joints

- Other targeted areas: Shoulders.
- Length of workout: 4 mins
- Time duration for resting periods: 5 -10 seconds in-between each set
- Estimated calorie burn: 12 calories.

Instructions

- Sit upright and comfortably in your chair.
- Turn your neck to the right as far as comfortable and hold for 5 seconds.
- Then relax for a second before turning it towards the left as far as comfortable and hold for 5 seconds.
- Now, bring your right ear to your right shoulder and hold for 5 seconds. Then bring your left ear to your left shoulder and hold for 5 seconds. That's one rep.
- Complete 3 sets of 5 reps.

Level up: To increase the stretch, hold on to your chair seat when performing the side-bends.

Precautions

- Bend your neck only in the pain-free range. If you feel any dizziness when bending your neck, stop the exercise.
- Try to keep your shoulders still when turning your head.
- Make sure you are bringing your ear to your shoulder and not the other way around.

Shoulder Circles

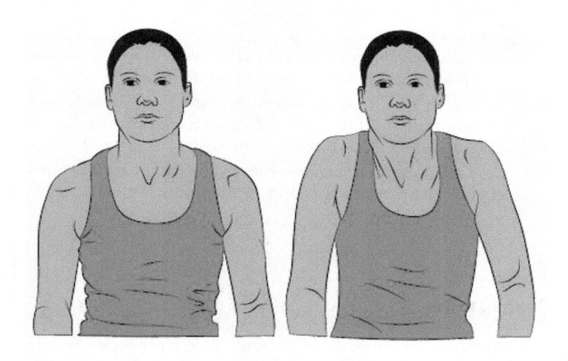

82. Shoulder Circles

Shoulder circles are dynamic stretches that gradually increase the range of motion of your shoulder joints. They also assist in keeping your rib muscles flexible.

- Other targeted areas: Arms, upper back.
- Length of workout: 4 mins
- Time duration for resting periods: 5 -10 secs in-between each set.
- Estimated calorie burn: 15 calories.
- Instructions
- Sit tall and comfortably in your chair with your elbows bent and fingertips placed on top of your shoulders.
- Keep your ribs lifted, as you slowly circle your shoulders 5 times forward and then circle 5 times backward. That's one set. Perform 2 more sets.
- To make it easier, imagine you are using the pointed end of your elbow to draw a circle on the wall.

Level up: Try doing these motions while standing up. That way, you will also be improving your balance as well as your range of motion.

Precautions

- Try to maintain your elbows high as you draw circles with your shoulders.
- Breathe normally.

Shoulder Stretch

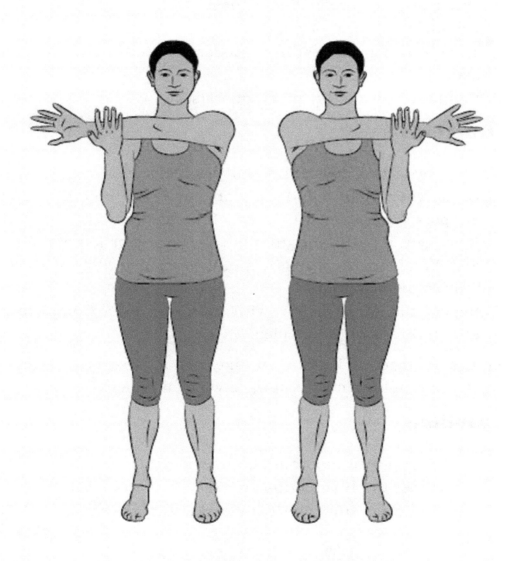

83. Shoulder Stretch

This exercise helps to stretch your shoulder, scapula, and other supporting muscles and joints in that area

- Other targeted areas: Neck, chest
- Length of workout: 4 mins
- Time duration for resting periods: 5 - 10 in-between each set
- Estimated calorie burn: 12 calories.

Instructions

- Start by sitting down with your back straight.
- Bring your right hand up onto your left shoulder and support your elbow with your left hand.
- Now, gently pull the right elbow toward your left shoulder and hold for 10 - 15 seconds. You'll definitely feel the stretch in your joints.
- Repeat the same motion with the other side. Complete 3 sets of 5 reps on both sides.

Level up: Instead of bending it like usual, keep your elbow straight when pulling it back toward your shoulder.

Precautions

- Try to keep your elbow at shoulder height.
- Remember to lift your ribs and keep your core tight.
- Stop if there is any joint pain during the movement

Chest Stretch

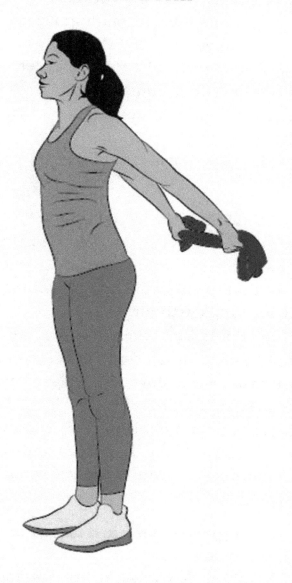

84. Chest Stretch

Performing chest stretches regularly will improve the mobility and flexibility in your upper chest and help the ventilation and functioning of your lungs. By stretching your chest muscles, you also get to maintain good rib mobility and improve your breathing.

- Other targeted areas: Shoulder muscles
- Length of workout: 4 mins
- Time duration for resting periods:5 -10 secs in-between each set.
- Estimated calorie burn: 12 calories.

Instructions

- Sit up and comfortably in your chair.
- Lift your arms and place your hands behind your head.
- Inhale as you gently bring your arms, neck, and shoulders back. At that point, you are stretching your chest and filling your lungs with air.
- Your chin should be tucked and your neck straight back.
- Now, hold that position for 1 to 3 seconds then exhale as you bring your arms down and relax. That's a rep!
- Complete 5 sets of 3 reps.

Level up: If you're up for a challenge, try leaning to the right and breathing out, while in the hands-behind-the-head position. Then in the following rep, lean to the left while breathing out.

Precautions

Ensure that you keep your ribs lifted as you breathe in and bring the neck and shoulders back.

Breathe deeply, all the way down to your abdomen.

Overhead Reach

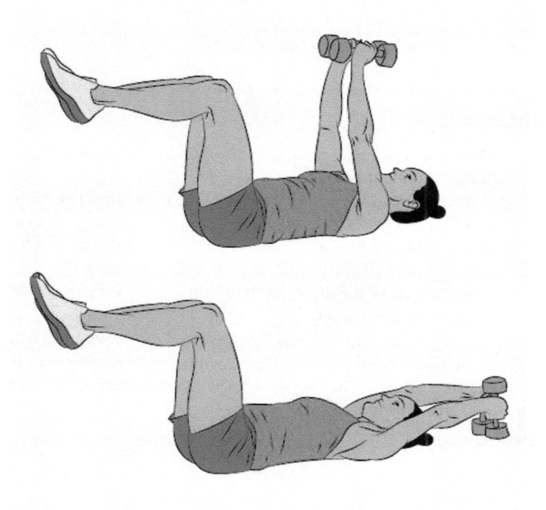

85. Overhead Reach

Overhead reach is another arm stretching exercise that strengthens your arms while giving you more range of motion and increasing your flexibility. These benefits will help you smoothly perform your daily functional movements.

- Other targeted areas: Shoulder muscles
- Length of workout: 4 mins
- Time duration for resting periods: 5 -10 secs in-between each set.
- Estimated calorie burn: 15 calories.

Instructions

- Begin sitting comfortably in your chair with your spine straight and ribs lifted.
- Take in a deep breath as you interlace your hands on your lap.
- Now exhale as you raise your arms overhead. Pause briefly after you have fully extended your arms overhead.
- Then return to the start position and repeat 5 times. Relax and go for 2 more sets.

Level up: To make this movement a little bit more complicated, lean to the right side with your hands overhead for a few seconds before lowering them. Then repeat on the left side during the next lift. Keep alternating like that.

Precautions

- Breathe normally through the nose and out through the mouth.
- Lift your arms only as high as is comfortable. Do not overdo it!

Reach Back

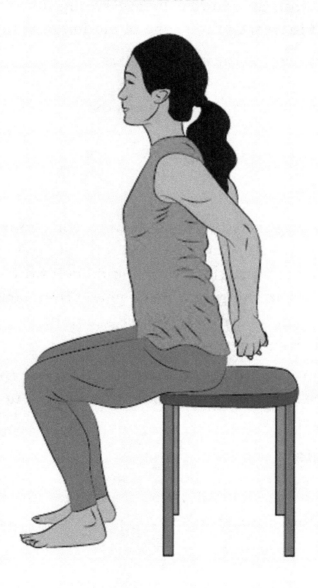

86. Reach Back

Like its name clearly states, the reach-back exercise improves your ability to reach behind like you are trying to reach back to hold onto an armrest before sitting down. The exercise stretches and increases the range of motion of your shoulders.

- Other targeted areas: Arms, chest.
- Length of workout: 4 mins
- Time duration for resting periods: 5 -10 secs in-between each set.
- Estimated calorie burn: 15 calories.

Instructions

- Stand upright with a chair behind you. Your back should be straight and your ribs lifted.
- Inhale as you interlace your hands behind your back.
- Breather out and gently move your arms backward.
- Pause, then return to the start position.
- Perform 3 sets of 5 reps.

Level up: Lean forward at the waist as you bring the arms back. This will force you to stretch your arms more, but be careful to not hyper-extend it.

Precautions

- Stop and take a break if you experience any pain.
- Don't move your arms too high.

Triceps Stretch

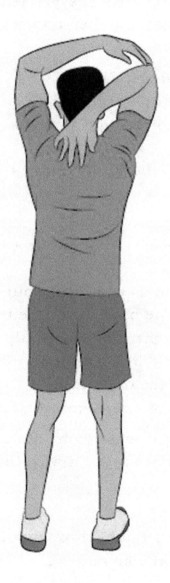

87. Triceps Stretch

Triceps stretches are great warm-up exercises that prepare your body for more intense exercises by increasing your blood circulation and delivering oxygen to muscles and the brain. Apart from this, it also stretches and improves the mobility of your triceps and shoulders.

- Other targeted areas: Chest
- Length of workout: 4 mins
- Time duration for resting periods: 5-10 secs in-between each set.
- Estimated calorie burn: 12 calories.

Instructions

- Begin by sitting in a chair while extending your left arm with your palm up.
- Tuck in your chin as you bring your left arm overhead and pat yourself on the back of your left shoulder.
- Now use your right hand to gently press your left elbow until a stretch is felt. Hold for 10 - 15 seconds. Then relax and repeat with the other arm.
- Complete 3 sets of 4 reps on each arm.

Level up: To increase the stretch, simultaneously raise your elbow higher as you try to press it with the opposite arm.

Precautions

- Keep your spine straight throughout the movements.
- Also, keep your abdominals tight.

Water Aerobics

Adding water aerobics is a great way to spice up your strength training program. In fact, it can serve as a great alternative on days you don't feel like doing traditional exercise. So, start getting your swimsuits and goggles ready as we examine these four effective water aerobics you can try as a senior.

Aqua jogging

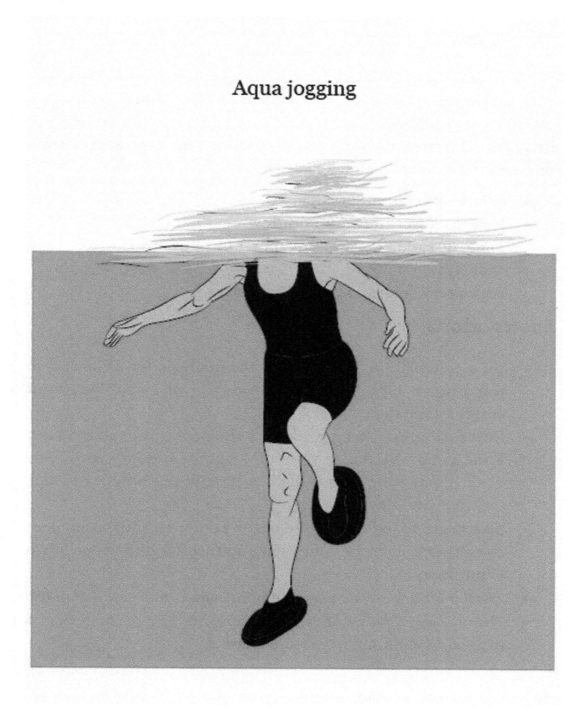

88. Aqua Jogging

Aqua jogging simply means you jog or run in water. Now, this low-impact aerobics is a great exercise to get your heart pumping and blood flowing throughout the body. It also helps in increasing flexibility and balance and, in the same way, decreasing bone and muscle loss.

- Other targeted area: Hips, knees
- Length of workout: 20 minutes
- Time duration for resting periods: 1 minute in-between each set.
- Estimated calorie burn: 230 calories.

Instructions

- Do a comfortable warm-up by the poolside for at least 3 to 5 minutes - high knees and jogging in place can work out correctly for them.
- Now rest a little, then wade into the pool until you're about waist deep. Visualize yourself jogging outdoors with your head lifted, your chin pulled-in, and your shoulder blades together and down.
- Now begin to jog to one end of the pool with your arms bent at a 90-degree angle and swinging through the water like a pendulum.
- Then jog back to the starting point again at a low intensity.
- That's 2 laps, so go ahead and perform 8 more laps. Rest a little, and then jog for 10 laps again.

Level up: To make this jogging a little more challenging, you can switch to jogging at high intensity.

Precautions

- If you are not comfortable with this jogging movement, you can walk back and forth in the pool or jog in a place using a swimming belt.
- Keep swinging your arms, and your back should be straight throughout these movements.

Leg Lifts

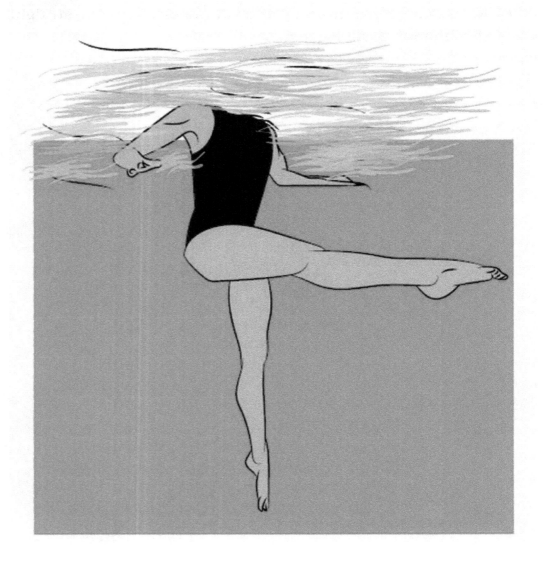

89. Leg Lifts

Taking advantage of the buoyancy and resistance of the water to perform leg lifts consistently helps to work and strengthen all of the leg muscles. This, in turn, improves your balance and cardio-vascular functions.

- Other targeted areas: Core, hip flexor and thighs.
- Length of workout: 6 mins
- Time duration for resting periods: 20 -30 secs in-between each set.
- Estimated calorie burn: 69 calories.

Instructions

- Stand in the pool and hold on to its edge.
- Now lift your right leg out to the side as far as you feel comfortable. Hold that position for 2 to 5 seconds before lowering it back down.
- Repeat 5 times before switching legs and performing the same routine on your left leg.
- Complete 2-3 sets of 5 reps on both legs.

Precautions

- If the hold feels uncomfortable or painful, lower your leg back down as soon as you lift it up. x Avoid rushing.

Flutter Kicking

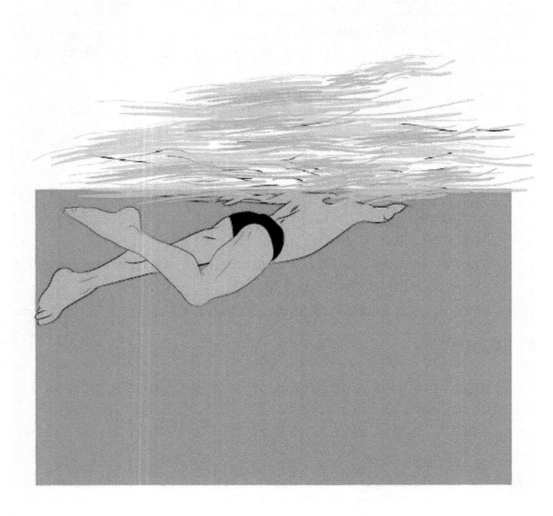

90. Flutter Kicking

Flutter kicking is a great low-impact cardio exercise for seniors. It basically targets and works your abdominal muscles and lower body, increasing strength and mobility in those areas. You will need a floating device like kickboard or pool noodle to keep your upper body afloat during this exercise.

- Other Targeted Areas: hip flexor, gluteus muscles.
- Length of workout: 6 mins
- Time duration for resting periods: 20 -30 secs in-between each set.
- Estimated calories burnt: 34 calories.

Instructions

- Get into the water and hold your floating device out in front of you, with your legs hanging towards the bottom of the pool.
- Once you are comfortable, begin to scissor kick your feet front-to-back rapidly across the pool.
- Your head and upper body should be kept afloat throughout the movement.
- As you kick, point your toes and keep your legs straight as comfortable.
- Repeat this movement 12 times, taking a break and then going ahead to do one more set of 12 reps.

Level up: As you begin to feel more comfortable in the water, you can try doing the exercise without the floating device.

Precautions

- Whichever you do this movement with or without a floating device, make sure you only kick at a steady tempo that doesn't weaken you too quickly but also gets the heart pumping.

Standing Water Push-Ups

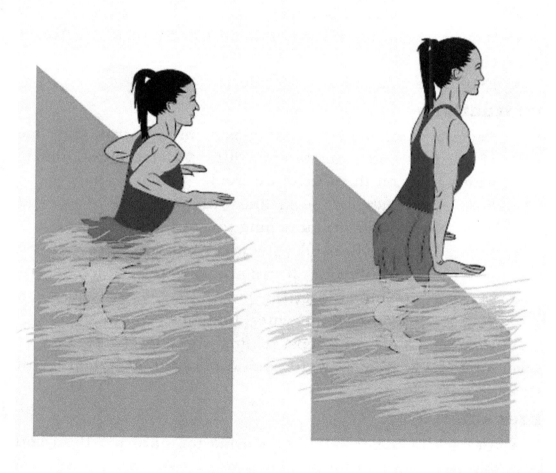

91. Standing Water Push-Ups

Often, the downside to traditional push-ups is that it involves putting too much pressure on most joints in your upper body. However, this water aerobics variation of standing push-ups cuts out those faults. It helps you increase strength and mobility in the muscles of your upper body.

- Other targeted areas: Arms, chest, shoulders.
- Length of workout: 5 mins
- Time duration for resting periods: 10 - 20 secs in between each set.
- Estimated calorie burn: 60 calories.

Instructions

- Begin by standing with your chest 2cm away from the edge of the pool and your hands a little wider than shoulder-width apart on the edge of the pool.
- Your elbows should be in line with your shoulders, and your feet shouldn't be touching the bottom of the pool.
- Inhale and slowly bend your arms as you lower yourself into the water till your elbows are bent to 90 degrees.
- Move as if you are getting out of the water and push yourself back out of the water. Exhale as you push up.
- Complete 3 sets of 4 reps, resting when necessary.

Level up: Make your upward and downward arm movement slower.

Precautions

- Be careful not to push your arms too hard mostly if you haven't figured out your limits.
- To reduce the strain on your arms during the push-ups, you can add a small jump.

- Keep your shoulders down, and avoid locking your elbows.

Arm Curls

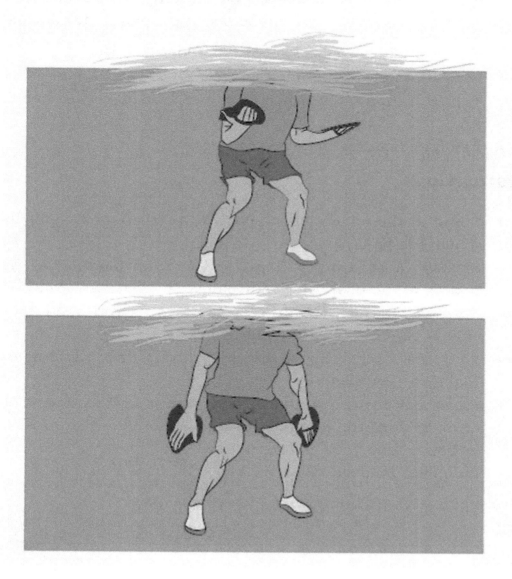

92. Arm Curls

The technique of this arm curl exercise still remains the same as the traditional one. However, the resistance of the water will work your muscles harder as you move them up and down. To perform this exercise, you will be needing a pair of dumbbells!

- Other targeted areas: Triceps, shoulders, chest.
- Length of workout: 5 mins
- Time duration for resting periods: 5 secs in-between each set.
- Estimated calorie burn: 60 calories.

Instructions

- Stand in the middle of the pool with the water dumbbells weights in your arms.
- Stretch those arms straight to the side, parallel to the bottom of the pool, with your palms facing downwards.
- Now, slowly push the dumbbells down as you bend your elbows together toward your armpits.
- Your shoulders should be still during this movement. Exhale as you bend.
- Pause for about 2 seconds, and then gently extend your arms back to the original position. Take in a deep breath as you extend your elbows.
- Complete 2-3 sets of 5 reps.

Level up: Switch to dumbbells of heavier weight.

Precautions

- Only from your shoulders to your lower body should be submerged in the water.
- Water weights are not mandatory. If you will be putting yourself at risk with the extra resistance, then ditch it and just repeat this exercise with you just clenching your fist.

Chair Yoga

Chair yoga is a highly beneficial low-impact form of yoga for seniors of any fitness level. All you need is an armless, stable chair and comfortable clothing that isn't too tight or baggy.

Overhead Stretch

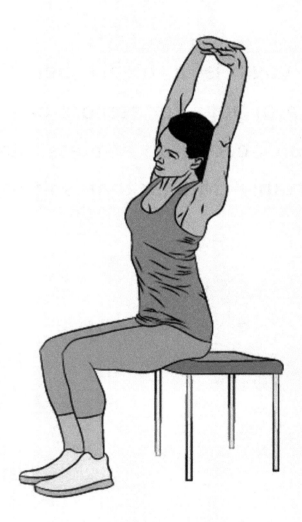

93. **Overhead stretch**

These exercises basically help you relieve your joint pains and improve your flexibility, blood circulation, and balance.

- Other targeted areas: Shoulders, back.
- Length of workout: 4 mins
- Time duration for resting periods: 10 - 20 secs in-between each set.
- Estimated calorie burn: 24 calories.

Instructions

- Get seated with your front-facing forward, your back straight, and your arms down by your sides.
- Keep your core tight as you take a long, deep breath in and slowly stretch your arms upward to the ceiling. Go as high as comfortable.
- Hold this position for about 5- 20 seconds, and lower your arms back downward. Make sure you do with a long exhale.
- Do 2 sets of 8-10 reps.

Level up: If you are up for a challenge, try using dumbbells to create extra resistance.

Precautions

- Keep your spine neutral throughout the entire movement.
- Do not over-extend your arms.

Seated Cow Stretch

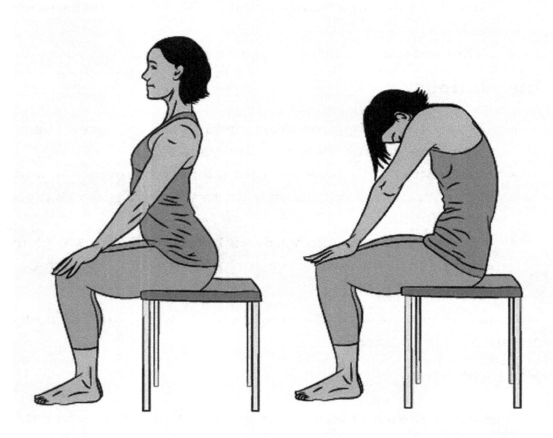

94. Seated Cow Stretches

This exercise is a yoga essential that helps ease pain in your spine and improve blood circulation in the discs in your back.

- Other targeted area: Core
- Length of workout: 5 mins
- Time duration for resting periods:
- Estimated calorie burn: 35 calories.

Instructions

- Get seated at the edge of your chair with your back as straight.
- Engage your core muscles and take in a deep breath as you gently arch your back as far as it is comfortable.
- Maintain that position for 3 to 5 breaths. Then bring your back to its original position.
- Complete 3 sets of 5 reps.

Precautions

- Remember that this exercise is supposed to be fun and comfortable, so stop when it begins to worsen.

Seated Cat Stretch

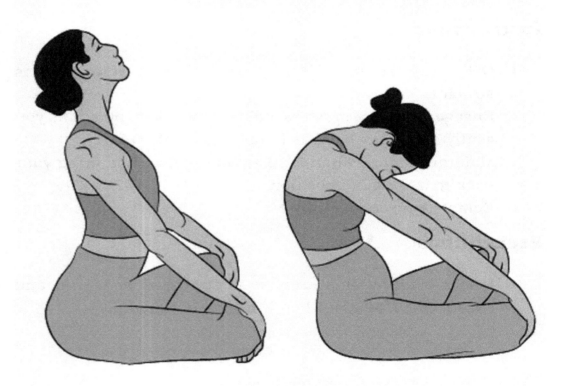

95. Seated Cat Stretches

This is the twin of the seated cow stretch movement. Often, they are combined as one. It is also useful for building a healthy spine.

- Other targeted areas: Abdominals, shoulders.
- Length of workout: 4 mins
- Time duration for resting periods: 5 secs in-between each set.
- Estimated calorie burn: 28 calories.

Instructions

- Begin by sitting on the edge of the chair with your spine in a neutral position.
- Now for the "cat" position, your shoulders should be directly above your hips as your back curves into a forward arch.
- Hold this position for 3 to 5 breaths before returning to your original seated position. That's one rep.
- Perform 3 sets of 5 reps, resting when necessary.

Level up: Deepen the intensity by drawing your navel in as firmly as possible during the pose.

Precautions

- This stretch should always be pain-free. So, if you feel any pain, gently back out.

Seated Mountain Pose

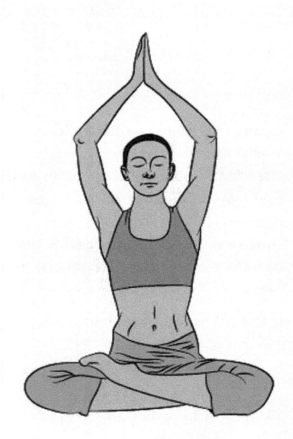

96. Seated Mountain Pose

The seated mountain pose is perfect for stretching your upper body's muscles, especially your trunk and shoulders. It helps relieve your joints of stress and strengthens them instead. As you stretch, your body is supposed to look like a mountain.

- Other targeted areas: Waist, hamstrings.
- Length of workout: 8 mins.
- Time duration for resting periods: 30-40 secs in-between each set.
- Estimated calorie burn: 56 calories

Instructions

- Sit comfortably in a sturdy chair with your back straight.
- Stretch your hands forward and interlock the fingers.
- With your hands and interlocked fingers still stretched in front of you, turn your palms outward.
- Now slowly raise the hands above your head, at the same time turning your palms upwards towards the roof.
- Make sure to align your head, trunk, and hands in a straight line as your Gaze straight ahead in a relaxed way.
- Breathe normally and make sure both your upper and lower body are stable. x Remain in this position for about 10 secs -30 secs as long as comfortable.
- To return to the original position, gently turn the palm inwards and bring down the hands. Release the interlocked fingers and let your palms rest on the thighs.
- Complete 4 sets of 3 reps

Precautions

- If you experience aching in your hands or shoulders at any position, make sure you can release the pose and take a break.
- Relax the whole upper body while keeping it straight and firm through the movement.

Seated Twist

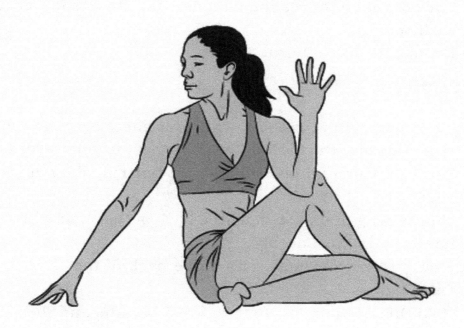

97. Seated Twist

This twisting exercise is a safe way to improve the flexibility of the spine, shoulders, and hips. It also keeps the joints in those areas very active, which indeed is a helpful necessity for seniors

- Other targeted areas: Neck, upper back, and arms.
- Length of workout: 4 mins
- Time duration for resting periods: 10 - 20 secs in-between each set.
- Estimated calorie burn: 28 calories.

Instructions

- Sit sideways in your chair, with your knees over the chair's right side and the back of the chair next to your right arm.
- Your back should be straight and not rested against the chair.
- Maintaining that pose, hold the back of the chair with both hands and inhale deeply.
- Slowly turn your body toward the back of the chair while exhaling.
- Hold this position for three to five 5 breaths and then turn back to your original position with the same control level.

Precautions

- Twist your body only within the range of comfort

Using Pilates

Pilates movement is a gentle strength-training exercise that has proven to be quite a useful tool for seniors looking to increase their physical strength and flexibility levels.

Mermaid Movement

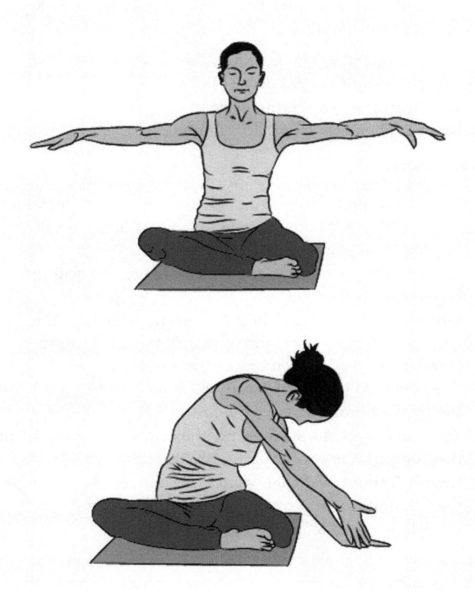

98. Mermaid Movement

This exercise is a Pilates mat exercise that lengthens your side body and provides inner body flow. It also helps in keeping the scapula muscle settled in your back.

- Other targeted areas: Obliques, shoulders, inner thighs
- Length of workout: 5 mins
- Time duration for resting periods:
- Estimated calorie burn: 20 calories.

Instructions

- Start by sitting on your mat with both of your legs folded to the left side. Make sure the back foot is flat on the floor to protect your knee.
- Also, place your right hand on the floor; this will give the boy support when you sit up.
- While keeping the left shoulder down and away from your ear, extend your left arm straight up and lengthen the spine as the body stretches to the side.
- The opposite (support) hand will move farther away from the body to increase the stretch
- To return back to start, send the left sit bone down and then engage the core to bring the torso up.
- Repeat 3 times and then switch the other side to complete the full movement.
- Complete 2 sets of 3 reps on each side.

Level up: As you become more comfortable with this stretch, you may try performing an arm circle with your upper arm at the top of the stretch.

Precautions

- Do not let your ribs pop forward as you curve to the side.
- Avoid arching your back or raising your shoulders.

Leg Circle

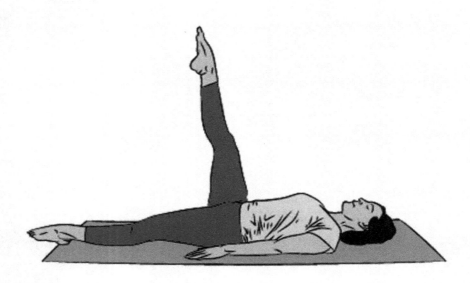

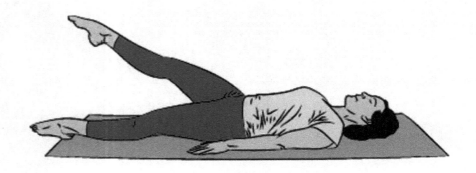

99. Leg Circle

Leg circles are classical Pilates mat exercise that is very effective for increasing your core strength and improving pelvic stability.

- Other targeted areas: Abdominal muscles, quads, hamstrings
- Length of workout: 8 mins
- Time duration for resting periods: 40- 1 minute's break in-between each set.
- Estimated calorie burn: 30 calories.

Instructions

- Lie on your back with your legs extended on the floor, arms by your sides.
- Draw in your abdominal muscles and stabilize your pelvis and shoulders.
- Now slowly pull your left knee in towards your chest and then extend it straight towards the roof.
- Cross that extended leg up and over the body, such that it angles up toward the opposite shoulder and over your right leg.
- Exhale and then lower the leg down towards the center line in a circling motion.
- Exercise control. You gently carry the open leg out to the side and then sweep it around back to center at your starting position.
- Perform two to three circles in this direction, then reverse by exhaling and then reaching your extended leg out to the side and then circling back toward and over the body.

- Stretch appropriately before switching legs. Do that by climbing your hands up your left leg to hold the ankle. Hold the position for two full breath cycles, gently pulling the leg closer and closer to you.
- Then repeat the first four steps on the opposite leg and finish with another stretch.
- Perform 2 sets of 5 reps on each leg.

Level up: Increase the size of the circle you make with your leg, and also try incorporating a resistance band into this exercise.

Precautions

- Keeping your shoulders and pelvis stable more important than making big circles with your legs.

Side Circles

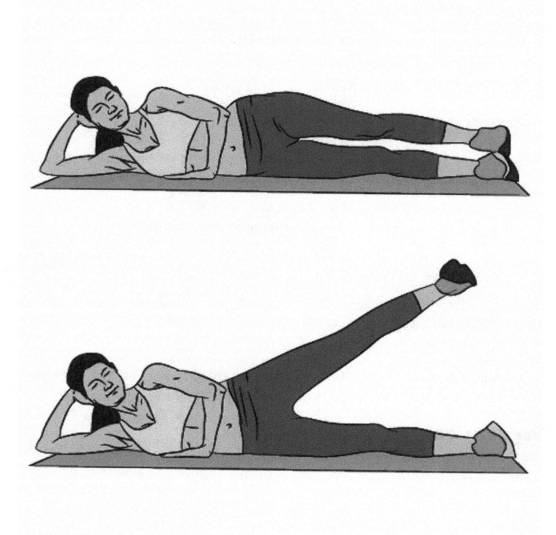

100. Side Circles

Just like the leg circles, this exercise also improves hip joint flexibility and lower body balance.

- Other targeted areas: Quadriceps, glutes.
- Length of workout: 5 mins
- Time duration for resting periods: 20 - 30 secs in-between each set.
- Estimated calorie burn: 25 calories.

Instructions

- To perform the side circle movement, lay on your left side and extend your leg towards the ceiling.
- Still maintaining that pose and engaging your core, slowly move your extended counterclockwise in small circles.
- Draw 2-3 circles and then reverse and move your leg clockwise to draw about 2-3 small circles.
- Gently lower your leg and switch to your right sides, repeating the same motions.
- Complete 2 sets of 4-6 reps on each leg.

Level up: Try increasing the size of the circle you draw with your legs. You can also add an elastic band to increase the resistance.

Precautions

- Only go as high as you feel comfortable.

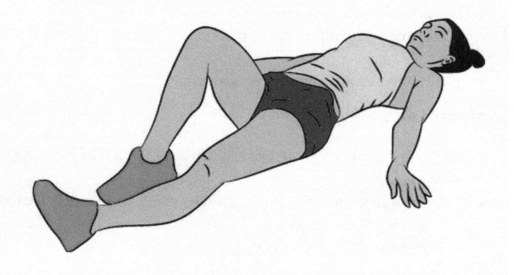

101. Foot Slides

Performing the foot slides pilates movement helps to activate and strengthen your deep core muscles and your hamstrings. By doing this, also aids in increasing your pelvic stability and balance.

- Other targeted areas: Ankle, knee.
- Length of workout: 4 mins
- Time duration for resting periods: 5 secs in-between each set
- Estimated calorie burn: 16 calories.

Instructions

- Begin by lying on your back with your knees bent and your core tight.
- Take a deep breath in and slowly slide your right foot out along the floor. Imagine that you're dragging your heel through sticky mud. That should make it easy.
- Keep the pelvis still and back relaxed throughout.
- Then exhale and slowly return to the starting position.
- Perform 3 sets of 5 reps on each leg.

Level up: You may add a 2-to-5-pound ankle weight to your leg.

Precautions

- Avoid lying on the bare floor; use a yoga mat or any comfortable mat.

90 Days Strength Training Exercise

Day 1 Triceps Stretch Biceps Curl Finger Bends Pelvic tilt	Day 2 Shoulder Circles Overhead stretch Finger Lifts Dumbbell Bench Press	Day 3 Step up Leg swings Knee extensions
Day 4 Seated Twist Lat Pull with Band Shoulder and Upper Back Stretch	Day 5 Tai Chi 8 forms Mermaid movement	Day 6 Upright Rows Wall Angels Neck rotation stretch
Day 7 Wall Push-Ups Forward punches Shoulder Rolls	Day 8 Lower back stretch Bent-Over Row Seated Twist Reverse Flyers	Day 9 Triceps Extension Lying hip bridges Wrist Stretches Good Mornings
Day 10 Chair Squat Sit to Stand Reach back Seated Marching on the spot	Day 11 Neck Side Stretch Shoulder Overhead Press Assisted Finger abductions stretch Hip Abductions	Day 12 Hamstring/Calf Stretch Bird dog Qigong knee rotation Wall slides
Day 13 Triceps stretch Seated Cow stretches Seated Cat stretch Ball Tap	Day 14 Chest Squeeze with Med Ball Triceps extension Ball squeezes Ball Tap	Day 15 Bicep curls Hand Open/Closes Bent Knee Raise Side Leg Raise Toe Raises
Day 16 Wall Angels Neck Rotation Squat Curl Knee Lift Quadriceps stretch Ankle Circles	Day 17 Chest stretches Chest Squeeze with Med Ball Mid-Back Extension Hip Abductions	Day 18 Finger Marching Standing Side Reach Shoulder Shrugs Overhead reach
Day 19 Triceps stretch	Day 20 Reverse Flyers	Day 21 Quadruped Opposite

Diagonal Shoulder Raise Hip Marching Toe Raise	Wall Slides Shoulder Overhead Press Knee Thrusters	Arm and Leg Balance Quadriceps Stretch Leg circles
Day 22 Rock the boat Seated twist Mid-Back Extension Ball squeezes	Day 23 Forward punches Aqua jogging Arms curls Standing water pushups	Day 24 The Basic Bridge Side circles Side-lying hip bridges
Day 25 Wall Slides Knee Curl Quadriceps stretch	Day 26 Step-Ups Aqua jogging Arms curls	Day 27 Reach back Seated Marching on the Spot Mid-back extension
Day 28 Single leg deadlift Quadriceps stretch Knee curls	Day 29 Lower Back Stretch Around the Clock Dumbbell Bench Press	Day 30 Bird Dog Leg Swings Hamstring/Calf Stretch
Day 31 Single-Leg deadlifts Rock the boat Leg Swings	Day 32 Jog in place Standing water push-ups Leg Lifts	Day 33 Reverse flyers Seated mountain pose Single-Leg Deadlifts
Day 34 Chest and Arm Stretch Back Leg Raise Side Leg Raise	Day 35 Shoulder Rolls Chair Dip Sit to Stand	Day 36 Seated mountain pose Back Leg Raise Reach back
Day 37 Forward punches Wrist radial Lat Pull with Band	Day 38 Thumb Flexion Ball Squeezes Forward punches	Day 39 Qigong knee rotation exercise Hip extensions Wall Angels
Day 40 Shoulder Stretch Shoulder Shrug Elbow flexion	Day 41 Overhead Reach Lying hip bridges Foot slides	Day 42 Chest Squeeze with Med Ball Triceps stretch Shoulder circles
Day 43 Step-Ups Overhead stretch Mermaid Movement	Day 44 Lat Pull with Band Seated Twist Shoulder and Upper Back Stretch	Day 45 Chest Stretch Kneeling Shoulder Tap Push Up Standing Side Reach
Day 46	Day 47	Day 48

The Basic Bridge Leg Circles Lower Back Stretch	Tai Chi 24 Forms Movement Qigong Knee Rotation Exercise	Hip extension Knee Thrusters Ankle Circles
Day 49 Hip Abductions Tai Chi 8 Forms Dumbbells Bench Press	Day 50 Jog in a place Standing water pushups Leg lifts	Day 51 Step-Ups Reverse Flyers Shoulder circles
Day 52 Mermaid Movement Diagonal Shoulder Raise Pelvic tilt	Day 53 Seated Mountain Pose Shoulder Press Lying Down Lying hip bridges	Day 54 Hip extensions Chair Squat Rock the boat
Day 55 Lat Pull with band Chest stretch Dumbbells Bench Press	Day 56 Chest and Arm Stretch Bicep curls Tai Chi 8 Forms Movement	Day 57 Finger Marching Overhead Reach Elbow flexion
Day 58 Mid-Back Extension Side circles Lying hip bridges	Day 59 Forward punches Upright Rows Knee curls	Day 60 Shoulder Shrug Neck Rotation Overhead stretch
Day 61 Quadriceps stretch Aqua jogging Water Arms curls	Day 62 Step-Ups Diagonal Shoulder Raise Quadruped Opposite Arm and Leg Balance	Day 63 Triceps extension Chest squeeze with Med Ball Standing Side Reach
Day 64 Jog in a place Diagonal Shoulder Raise Pelvic tilt	Day 65 Tai Chi 24 forms Elbows pronation Elbow Side Extensions	Day 66 Seated cow stretches Seated cat stretches Lower back stretch
Day 67 Standing Side Reach Sit to stand Chair Squat	Day 68 Mermaid Movement Shoulder rolls Shoulder stretch	Day 69 Side Hip Raise Leg swings Wall Slides
Day 70 Shoulder Press Lying Down Hip Abductions Basic bridge	Day 71 Tai Chi 8-Forms movement Seated Twist Seated Cow Stretch	Day 72 Shoulder and Upper Back Stretch Standing Water Push- ups Leg Lifts
Day 73 Step-Ups	Day 74 Triceps extension	Day 75 Qigong knee rotation

Back leg raise Bent knee raise	Assisted Finger Abductions Give the okay Make a "C"	exercise Quadriceps stretch Knee curls
Day 76 Triceps extension Chair squat Seated chair twist	Day 77 Mermaid Movement Tai Chi 8 forms	Day 78 Quadruped Opposite Arm and Leg Balance Leg Swings Toe Raises
Day 79 Finger Marching Triceps extension Overhead Reach	Day 80 Lat Pull with Band Seated Twist	Day 81 Shoulder and Upper Back Stretch Quadruped Opposite Arm and Leg Balance
Day 82 Ball Tap Side leg raise Around the clock	Day 83 Kneeling Shoulder Tap Push Up The basic bridge Seated mountain pose	Day 84 Finger Marching Give the okay Thumb flexion Wrist flexion
Day 85 Step-Ups Wall push-ups Wrist stretches Chest squeeze with Med Ball	Day 86 Biceps curls Shoulder shrugs Forward punches	Day 87 Leg swings One-legged Squat Ankle circles
Day 88 Standing side reach Shoulder circles Upright rows	Day 89 Forward punches Reach back Single-leg deadlift	Day 90 Jog in a place Aqua jogging Standing water pushups

Conclusion

Thank you for making it to the other end of this book. At this point, I'm sure that you have fully understood that as you grow older, an active life is more important than ever. Imagine how satisfying it would feel to move all your joints fluidly and without feeling any painful niggles that usually come with tight aging muscles and joints.

This book has equipped you with ALL the tools you need to not just regain your once-upona-time youthful strength but also to improve your flexibility, balance, and stability level in different parts of your upper and lower body.

Of course, there is a lot here to take in and do. But the primary key to your fitness growth and success is for you to keep it simple and stay consistent! Functional independence isn't regained in just a few days or weeks; you have to be resilient to get it! The best time to start was yesterday, but the second-best time is now!

References

Atkinson, D. (n.d.). Upper Arm Exercises You Can Do in the Pool. Retrieved from

https://primewomen.com/health/fitness/pool-arm-exercises/

Bowling, N. (2016). Wall Pushup Variations for A Strong Chest, Shoulders, and Back.

Retrieved from https://www.healthline.com/health/fitness-exercise/wall-pushups

Cordeau, B. (n.d.) How to Do: Lat Pulldown Loop Band. Retrieved from

https://www.skimble.com/exercises/41947-lat-pulldown-loop-band-how-to-do-exercise

East Wind Tai Chi Association. (n.d.). Tai Chi Forms. Retrieved from

http://www.itatkd.com/taichi-forms.html

Garofalo. M. P. (n.d.). Taijiquan 24 Form Yang Style. Retrieved from

https://www.egreenway.com/taichichuan/short.htm#Descriptions

Ghosh, A. (2017). Pilates for Seniors – The Complete Guide. Retrieved from

https://www.vivehealth.com/blogs/resources/pilates-for-seniors

Just Swim. (n.d.) Tone Your Body with Pool Edge Push-Ups. Retrieved from

https://www.swimming.org/justswim/pool-edge-push-ups/

Kenler, M. (2021) Banded Lat Pulldown: A Complete Guide | Form, Benefits & Alternatives. Retrieved from

https://www.anabolicaliens.com/blog/banded-lat-pulldown

Liang, H. (2015). Discover the Tai Chi 24 Forms. Retrieved from

https://ymaa.com/articles/2015/10/discover-the-tai-chi-24-form

Liang, H. (2016). Tai Chi 24-Form Movements. Retrieved from

https://ymaa.com/articles/2016/02/step-by-step-tai-chi-24-form

Lifeline. (n.d.). 14 Exercise for Seniors to Improve Strength and Balance. Retrieved from

   https://www.lifeline.philips.com/resources/blog/2018/07/14-exercises-for-seniors-toimprove-strength-and-balance.html

Lindberg, S. (2020). Benefits of Jogging and Tips to Get Going. Retrieved from

   https://www.healthline.com/health/aqua-jogging

Mansur, R. (2018). Do Bicep Curls for Seniors. Retrieved from

   https://weighttraining.wonderhowto.com/how-to/do-bicep-curls-for-seniors-254684/

More Life Health: Seniors. (n.d.) Bicep Curl Exercise. Retrieved from

   https://morelifehealth.com/bicep-curls

Nurse Next Door. (2020). 6 Easy and Safe Exercises for Seniors. Retrieved from

   https://www.nursenextdoor.com/blog/6-easy-and-safe-exercises-for-seniors/

Occhipinti, A. (2018). 3 Pilates Exercises to Help Seniors Improve Balance & Mobility. Retrieved from

   https://www.afpafitness.com/blog/pilates-exercises-help-seniorsimprove-balance-mobility

Ogle, M. (2020). How to Do Mermaid Sides Stretch in Pilates: Proper Form, Variations, and Common Mistakes. Retrieved from

   https://www.verywellfit.com/learn-mermaid-sidestretch-2704698

Ogle, M. (2020). How to Do Single Leg Circle in Pilates: Proper Form, Variations, and Common Mistakes. Retrieved from

   https://www.verywellfit.com/how-to-do-one-legcircle-2704673

Pizer, A. (2020) How to Do Cat-Cow Stretch (Chakravakasana) in Yoga. Retrieved from

   https://www.verywellfit.com/cat-cow-stretch-chakravakasana-3567178

Qiyas. (n.d.). Best Pool Exercises for Seniors: Legs, Knee, Arms, Core. Retrieved from

https://hydroactive.ca/pool-exercises-for-seniors/

Ratini, M. (2020). 10 Ways to Exercise Hands and Fingers. Retrieved from

https://www.webmd.com/osteoarthritis/ss/slideshow-hand-finger-exercises

Schrift, D. (n.d.) Upper Arm Exercise for Seniors and The Elderly. Retrieved from

https://eldergym.com/upper-arm-exercises/

Senior Lifestyles. (n.d.) Infographic: Top 10 Chair Yoga Position for Seniors. Retrieved from

https://www.seniorlifestyle.com/resources/blog/infographic-top-10-chair-yogapositions-for-seniors/

Shillington, P. (2017). Never Too Late: Building Muscles and Strength After 60. Retrieved from

https://baptisthealth.net/baptist-health-news/never-late-building-musclestrength-60/

Shou-Yu, L. (2012). Learning Tai Chi – The 24 and 48 Forms. Retrieved from

https://ymaa.com/articles/learning-tai-chi-the-24-and-48-forms

Talk Early, Talk Often. (n.d.). Exercise for Senior Citizens: Try Triceps Extensions for Aging Fitness. Retrieved from

http://www.talk-early-talk-often.com/exercise-for-seniorcitizens.html

The Middletown Home. (n.d.). The Benefits of Tai Chi for Seniors. Retrieved from

https://middletownhome.org/tai-chi-benefits-seniors/

Tummee. (n.d.). Chair Seated Twists. Retrieved from

https://www.tummee.com/yogaposes/chair-seated-twists

Waehner, P. (2019). Total Body Strength Workout for Seniors. Retrieved from

https://www.verywellfit.com/total-body-strength-workout-for-seniors-1230958

Williams, L. (2020). How to Do a Side Lateral Raise: Proper Form, Variations, and Common Mistakes. Retrieved from

https://www.verywellfit.com/side-lateral-raise-4588211

Willhoite, J. (2020). Punching Bag Workout Tips for Seniors Stress Relief. Retrieved from

https://seniorslifestylemag.com/health-well-being/punching-bag-workout-tips-forsenior-stress-relief/

BOOK 2

Strength Training After 40

A Practical Guide to Building and Maintaining a
Healthier, Leaner, and Stronger Body

Introduction

If you are over the age of 40 and are committed to getting into shape whether it's for the first time or you want to return to the physical condition of when you were younger, you have taken an important first step: the objective of this book is to help you attain a stronger, leaner body leading to better health and well-being, and to get you there safely and effectively with exercise routines and lifestyle improvements you can easily adopt and follow.

You are right to want to build a strong, lean body, exchanging fat for muscle mass, building strength and endurance, improving your health, and increasing your disease resistance. People over 40 can become strong and fit, but the exercise routines to get them there are not the same as when they were 20 or 25, Your body has changed, yet with the correct, scientifically evolved, and tested training techniques, you will be surprised how soon you will see and feel real progress.

You'll be impressed to know how many people over 40 who were not satisfied with their bodies and physical conditions have decided they would commit to shape up, do it right, and get the results they want. Their positive results include building lean muscle mass, getting more definition, reducing fat, especially around the belly, increasing energy and endurance, and feeling better about themselves. It can work for you as your state of mind will improve with a greater feeling of self-esteem, reduced anxiety, and a positive belief that anything is possible no matter your age.

What Are Your Fitness Goals?

Do you want to be proud when you look in a mirror and see muscles returning after being soft and hidden under a layer of flab? Or see that your potbelly has diminished as your abs become more defined? Are you among the two-thirds of Americans who are overweight or obese, and you want to lose the excess weight as an investment in your overall health and longevity?

Now that you are over 40, do you realize that has your cardiovascular health should be a priority? Do you know that heart disease becomes a risk as middle-age progresses? That heart attacks and strokes can be averted with the proper conditioning and dietary practices?

It's Up to You: Motivation and Commitment

Achievement of your muscle- and strength-building goals and attainment of real physical fitness are dependent upon the levels of your motivation and commitment. It's important to understand that you'll be exercising at least several days per week with resistance training that may involve lifting, pulling, and stretching, plus raising your heart rate for sustained periods through cardio, or aerobic, exercises. Be assured that with the training advice you receive here, these routines will not take up much time and are easy to learn with our instructions.

Ask yourself why you want to get into shape and achieve your physical fitness goals. What is motivating you? There is no right or wrong reason for your commitment. What matters is that you have the drive and tenacity to stay with it, starting from the initial first exercises, then gradually increasing to more intensive routines. You will not be alone as you join the many others who have recognized the value of middle-age strength training.

Resistance exercises can be performed in fitness centers or your home. You can do body calisthenics in a small easy-to-assemble home gym. You also can do them without dumbbells, barbells, cables, and machines. What matters most is not the equipment, but rather your commitment to follow the instructions and perform the exercises. Don't let yourself become one of those people who joins a fitness center, buys equipment, but never follows through. Good intentions are one thing; motivation and commitment are another.

This Book is Your Roadmap

This book will enable you to achieve your fitness goals. It recognizes the need to present the most effective exercise routines for you while respecting your age and current fitness level. Whether you are just turning age 40, or are well beyond, the benefits of resistance and cardiovascular conditioning are clinically proven to be beneficial at every age. Also, as you mature, good dietary practices take on added importance to your health and longevity

The motivations that ignite your desire to begin a strengthening and conditioning program need to be strong enough to keep you committed to turn physical fitness and muscle-building into an integral lifestyle component. That is why we are providing step-by-step training, options to fit your personal preferences, and the availability of where and how to train.

You Have the Time

Too often we hear the excuse, "I don't have time to work out," and this may be expressed by men and women at any age. The reality is they either are not motivated to get into a workout routine or deeply committed to keeping it going and making it part of their lifestyle. They have not accepted how essential their strength and fitness workouts are for their health and wellness, for how they look, and for how they feel. It takes inner psychological strength to face those weights and cables, treadmill or exercise bike at daybreak or before lunch or dinner.

No one ever ends a good workout session feeling it was a waste of time. On the contrary, they're pumped up by the satisfaction of lifting weights correctly, getting their heart rate up, and their arteries flowing along with the "high" that comes from the beta-endorphin hormones that vigorous exercise releases.

Exercises Targeted to Your Age

This book was written for you at a stage in your life when your physical condition and overall shape are not what they used to be. The exercises to build muscles, and get you into great shape, are not the same as those you did when you were younger. We've done the research to identify the types of exercises and routines that are best for you now. You will learn how to get started, which exercises are best to get you started, how often to train, when to rest and recover, and how to progress. You will learn the fundamental exercises for optimal results while avoiding complicated, potentially harmful exercises best left for professionals.

All strengthening exercises in this book are explained and demonstrated, so you will have no difficulties in learning how to perform the movements correctly.

As we age, our exercise needs evolve, too. Certain muscle groups need more attention to keep our guts flat, to help protect our backs from soreness and pain, to help us improve our balance, and to help prevent falls that can cause hip fractures and other serious injuries. Middle-age weightlifting may require a more careful selection of weights, movements, repetitions, and rest periods between sets. As you will see, the core of muscle building is hypertrophy, which is the breaking down of muscle fibers, and the subsequent repair and rebuilding. Rest is essential for this process to succeed. Our training plans consider all these factors so you don't have to worry about them.

Overview by Chapters

This book is organized to guide you through the nature of your body now that you have reached middle-age. It will show you that while your body is different than it was, you are still able to lift weights, use muscle-building equipment, and perform bodyweight calisthenics to build lean, well-defined muscle mass and grow stronger. You will be guided through cardiovascular exercises you can perform to get into great physical condition. Your diet will play an important role in your health and muscle-building, and the overriding principles are the motivation to start and the commitment to stay with it.

Chapter 1 will help you gain an appreciation of how your body has evolved and how at age 40 or older, it is not the same as it was at 20 or 25. Unless, of course, you've been working out continuously with progressively heavier weights, which most of us certainly have not been doing. The majority of us has become more sedentary: riding instead of walking and running, sitting instead of standing, and no longer lifting the weights and doing the calisthenics that kept our muscles firm and our bodies lean. Our bodies have followed our lead and slowed, leaving us with less lean muscle mass and more body fat, showing itself in a growing waistline. This adds up to you not being able to pick up where you left off and lift weights and do intense exercises like you used to.

Chapter 2 will convince you that your age is not a barrier to achieving ambitious musclebuilding goals. It's well established that you can build lean, strong muscles at age 40 and beyond. It's just a matter of performing the right exercises with the right weights and routines. Muscle and strength-building is a matter of applying scientific and effective principles that reduce the risk of injury while optimizing results in the shortest time. It is definitely not too late to get started, and now is an excellent time to make the commitment and start lifting.

Chapter 3 will reassure you of your ability to lift heavy weights despite what you might have heard. Being a middle-aged weightlifter does not mean you cannot lift heavy weights, or that heavier weights are for youngsters and you need to lighten up. Opinions are one thing, and experience and research are another. The evidence, based on extensive training and coaching, is that heavy weights are the way to go at middle-age. You will meet action-hero celebrities whom you admire and who will share workouts with you that helped propel them to superstar status. You will see that if your goal is to build lean, well-defined muscle mass, heavy weights are the right weights as long as they aren't too heavy.

Chapter 4 covers your exercise selection and recovery routine. You will be doing exercises with heavy weights, but they will not necessarily be the same exercises you performed when you were younger or that you see someone else doing at the fitness center. Some weightlifting exercises are safe for you at this age. Others that you may have once performed are now too risky and need to be avoided. Recovery time after hard exertion was important when you were younger to enable the hypertrophy rebuilding process to function, but now it's doubly important because, after age 40, hypertrophy takes longer and the risk of injury from overwork is greater. Your patience will be rewarded with results.

Chapter 5 is about commitment. With your metabolism gradually slowing down, the need for your commitment to physical fitness and building lean muscle intensifies. With age, you lose lean muscle mass at an increased rate each year. At the same time, your body increases its storage of excess energy as fat. Your gut shows that result as you wonder, "Where did my sixpack abs go?" This is when you need to look in the mirror and make the personal commitment to go the distance. Decide there will be no excuses to keep you from becoming a muscular, strong, physically impressive person who faces middle-age with confidence.

Chapter 6 is about the importance of a healthy diet. Your health, strength, and endurance depend on the fuel you ingest, the quality and types of foods you eat. As crucial as weightlifting is to build muscles and become stronger and more fit, your diet is even more influential. The carbohydrates, proteins, and fats in your diet need to be well-sourced from healthy, more natural, less processed food that provides the essential vitamins, minerals, and antioxidants that your body needs. There is a range of diets that you can consider, but we'll introduce you to one that is more than just a diet. It's a complete lifestyle overhaul with a wide range of delicious foods that you will love without having to count calories. In recognizing that our diet plays a key role in building muscle and keeping off fat, we'll help you cut through all the dietary misinformation and embrace a lifelong dietary practice rather than a fad diet that will come and go. There are fundamentals of nutrition that you will learn to follow.

Chapter 7 will address and debunk the misconceptions that can interfere with your commitment and motivation. You'll discover that your workouts can take less time than you think. That you can put real effort and intensity into your exercise routines and get more out of your investment in time and energy. You will get a new perspective on running, walking, and other proven forms of cardiovascular conditioning, and you'll understand how diet and exercise can work synergistically to get your weight where it belongs, to help strengthen your immune system, and to prevent diseases.

About the Author

CJD Fitness founder Baz Thompson is a CYQ Master Personal Trainer who has helped hundreds of people like you achieve their fitness goals. Baz works with professional athletes in world-renowned fitness facilities as well as coaching global executives and almost everyone in between, including people of all ages who fly in from around the world to benefit from his personal training. His certifications include Kettlebell Concepts, PROnatal Fitness Pre- and Post-Natal, and TRX Level 2.

Baz realizes that too many people approach middle-age with a sense of frustration about lifting weights, building muscle, and getting back into shape. But, Baz says it doesn't have to be that way: it's not too late to get started in a well-planned weightlifting and conditioning program. If you have the motivation to take charge of your physical fitness and get into shape, to build lean muscle mass and get rid of fat, to revitalize your cardiovascular conditioning and boost your self-esteem, and feel absolutely great about yourself and how you look, this is the one roadmap that you need. This professional, step-by-step coaching on exercise and diet will help you achieve all of your fitness goals after age 40 and well beyond.

"I am excited to be your trainer, coach, and advisor on this journey to achieving strong, lean muscles that are well defined and functional as well as helping you lower your body fat level and bring your weight into a healthy range. You will be joining the hundreds of people I have trained and helped achieve their fitness and strength goals at a time in their lives when they thought it was too late for them. It was not too late for them, and it is not too late for you" – Baz Thompson (2020).

Are you ready? Let's get your fitness education and training started!

Chapter 1

Your Body Has Evolved

A recently published online article in WebMD (2020) underscores the importance of exercise during middle-age and makes the point that while you no longer have the body of a 20-yearold, exercise that makes you stronger and gets you into shape is more important now than when you were younger. Being stronger and more physically fit is essential to maintaining a good quality of life and keeping your independence as you mature.

The benefits of weight training and other forms of resistance exercises, along with keeping up aerobically through cardiovascular training, are considerable for those of us who are over 40, 50, or more.

➤ Muscles burn more calories compared to body fat even when you are at rest. This can offset the effects of middle-age slowing of your metabolism and make it easier to keep extra pounds from adding up.

➤ Consistent exercise is credited with helping to slow or prevent the onset of life-threatening diseases that may begin in middle-age, including hypertension, strokes, atherosclerosis and other types of heart disease, diabetes, osteoporosis, and certain types of cancer.

➤ Strength and fitness training are believed to slow the progression of Alzheimer's disease and other forms of dementia as well as the cognitive decline that slows down the brain's usual sharpness.

These are the concerns that we'll address in this chapter and will guide you in how to know yourself, build up yourself, and protect yourself.

Know Thyself

The ancient Greek aphorism, "Know thyself," is engraved as a maxim on the Temple of Apollo in Delphi, and it is an appropriate prequel for your strength training over age 40. As you ramp up your motivation and commitment, it is important to pause for a moment and take stock of who you are at this point in your life.

Your body is no longer that of a teenager or young adult because with the years come physical changes. Some are due to inevitable wear and tear from life's stresses while others are results of the aging process. Your muscles are gradually atrophying, ligaments, joints, and tendons are not as flexible, and your resilience is slower, meaning it takes you longer to recover after hard exertion. Your body shape may have changed, and your midsection may be getting larger.

Other, more subtle changes may be quietly working behind the scenes and slowing down your metabolism, which is the overall rate of your body's functioning.

All of this adds up to you not being able to pick up where you left off and lift weights and do intense exercise like you used to. But it is certainly not too late to return to a full exercise and fitness program focusing on weightlifting.

You can slow the aging process through exercise and diet, rebuild lost muscle mass, build new, larger muscles, and gain appreciable strength. That's what this book is all about: restoring your body to earlier strength, building new muscle mass, increasing flexibility, getting your weight down, and keeping your arteries clear to slow the onset of cardiovascular disease.

Benchmarking 1: Measuring Up

Assessing your current condition is the best way to objectively determine where you are physically right now before beginning your weight training and overall physical improvement program. The first stage of this benchmarking assessment is how you look and measure up.

The mirror, the scale, and the tape measure are impartial judges of how well you are doing and can help you set goals for where you want to go. Begin by looking in the mirror while in your underwear and objectively consider how you look. Don't be hard on yourself; just take an assessment of where you are now and consider it a benchmark, a starting point. Check out your upper arms: how firm and defined are the biceps upfront, and the triceps behind? Are your chest muscles, the pectorals or "pecs," starting to sag? Next, is there any definition to your abdominal muscles or sign of the famous "six-pack" of well-developed abs? Finally, how about your thighs and calves? If you stand sideways and lower yourself partially in a half deep knee bend, can you see any definition in your legs?

Make a mental note of what you see or, even better, write it down.

Step on the scale, preferable before breakfast in your underwear, barefoot, and at the same time and conditions each day. After noting your weight on the first day, go online and check your Body Mass Index (BMI), which is based on your height and weight. A BMI of 18.5 to 24.9 is normal, 25 to 29.5 is overweight, and 30 and higher is considered obese. Don't be upset if you are overweight or obese; two-thirds of American adults are, but make a commitment that you will work to get that weight down close to the normal range. It's important:

> According to the National Heart, Lung, and Blood Institute (2020), the higher a person's BMI, the greater the risk for diseases, including type 2 diabetes, heart disease, high blood pressure, respiratory problems, gallstones, and certain types of cancer.

Be patient: it took time to gain the extra weight, so it will take time to get rid of it. Your diet will play a key role along with exercise, so be sure to give the upcoming chapter on diet your fullest attention.

The tape measure is the last appearance and physical measurement benchmark, and like the scale, it is completely objective. It doesn't lie, exaggerate, or coddle you.

> Measure your waistline at the level between the top of your hip bones and naval, pulling the tape firmly but not too tight. Exhale just before you measure. Be aware that the measure for a man should not exceed 40 inches (102 cm), and for a woman, it's 35 inches (89 cm).

Beyond those measurement limits, professionals say there's too much belly fat, and that can interfere with numerous bodily functions. It also can possibly lead to the same diseases as an elevated BMI.

Benchmarking 2: Measuring Strength

The second phase of your benchmarking assessment is to see how much strength you have. A licensed physical trainer can run you through a series of measurements with different exercises and may even take a calculation of body fat and lean muscle percentages.

But you can take your own simple strength measurement by dropping down and seeing how many **push-ups** you can do. Start in a plank position, legs extended to the rear, arms fully extended shoulder-width apart, and your back level (no sagging or arching). Lower down fully so your nose or chest touches the floor, raise back up to the starting position, and repeat as many times as you can. Don't race: take about three seconds for each down-and-up cycle. Write down your total.

If you have access to a pull-up or chin-up bar, count how many pull-ups you can do (a pullup is with your palms facing forward). Place your hands shoulder-width apart and pull up fully, lower all the way down ((not too fast), and repeat as many times as you can in good form (no half-ways). When you're done, write down the total. Or, if you can use dumbbells, determine the maximum weight you can curl eight to 10 times maximum. A curl is raising the dumbbells from the arms-lowered position up to your shoulders, then slowly lowering back down.

As your weight training program progresses, you can periodically repeat these exercises and measure your improvements.

Fitness, Health, Longevity

Your motivation to get into, or get back into, weightlifting and other exercises to gain strength in middle-age is based, at least in part, on how you want to look and feel. You want to see a well-built body in the mirror with visibly larger, defined muscles and a flatter gut. You want to feel the muscles expanding under your skin at the end of your workouts as blood rushes to the hard-working muscle cells and fibers in the "pumping iron" effect. You want more energy, more bounce to your step, more endurance to keep you going longer. You want to look and feel fit. You want to be stronger.

These are the motivating factors that will get you started on your weight and strength-building program. They hopefully will be enough to keep you going because achieving your fitness goals will take time and effort.

To further reinforce your commitment, let's pick up on what was mentioned above in the discussion of benchmarking: the health aspects of getting in shape and staying in shape, and getting your weight down and keeping it down.

More Life to Your Years

There's an expression that was popular among long-distance runners and has spread to the weightlifting and fitness community overall:

> ➤ *"Working out and staying in shape will add more life to your years and may even add more years to your life."*

In other words, your commitment to building muscle and getting into good cardiovascular condition definitely will make every day richer and more vibrant and may also help you to live longer. All in all, that's not a bad deal. It gives you something to work for, to invest time and energy in, and stay with over the long term.

According to the Mayo Clinic (2020), regular exercise can improve health and manage the symptoms of chronic illnesses that are long-term, limit activities, and interfere with a normal lifestyle. Given the importance of exercise in preventing heart disease, it is covered separately in the following section.

Everyday activities. Strength training with weightlifting not only improves muscle strength and increases endurance, but makes daily activities easier to do and slows the decline in muscle strength related to disease. Every day, we are lifting, carrying, standing, walking, crouching, bending, and generally challenging our muscles, joints, bones, and tendons as well as pushing our circulatory and respiratory systems as we work our hearts and lungs during exertion. The better the state of our physical condition, the easier the work we do will be, and when we're in good shape, we feel better.

Joint stability. Flexibility exercises can help you regain an optimal range of motion by providing stability to your joints to enhance their functionality, and the risk of falls can be reduced with stability exercises. Weightlifting and other resistance exercises, when done correctly, will increase stability and flexibility and will further help by strengthening the muscles that support the joints. For example, by strengthening the quadriceps muscles at the front of our thighs, we can help control the kneecap and knee socket, preventing excess motions that can wear away the cartilage that lubricates and cushions the knees.

Diabetes. Regular exercise can lower the risk of adult-onset type 2 diabetes by enabling insulin to lower blood sugar levels more effectively. For those already with type 2 diabetes, resistance exercise with weightlifting, along with aerobics, can reduce the risk of heart disease.

Type 2 diabetes is often associated with obesity, so the weight reduction benefits of exercise can directly reduce the risks and symptoms of diabetes.

Weight control. Physical activity can help you control your weight and boost your energy because weightlifting burns calories as does cardiovascular training. However, exercise alone does not optimize weight loss; it is the combination of diet and exercise that is most effective. In a later chapter, we'll examine how diet and exercise combined can make the greatest effects in getting those excess pounds off and keeping them off.

Arthritis. Exercise has been found t0 reduce joint pain, maintain muscle strength in arthritisaffected joints, and reduce stiffness in joints, resulting in improved quality of life and physical function even for those who have been suffering from arthritis for years. Those with arthritis symptoms should choose low-impact exercise. Any weightlifting that puts extra pressure on joints may require modifying certain movements to reduce the strain.

Asthma. The heavy, deeper breathing associated with weightlifting and all intensive exercise appears to help reduce the severity and frequency of asthma attacks. The depth of breathing during exercise, combined with increased blood circulation and oxygen delivery, may strengthen the lungs and air sacs where oxygen is transferred to the bloodstream. The deep breathing performed during intense exercise also strengthens the diaphragm muscle, which controls breathing by facilitating inhaling and exhaling.

Back pain. Abdominal and core-challenging resistance exercises strengthen the muscles around your spine, and these exercises may help reduce back pain symptoms. Also, low-impact aerobic exercises, performed regularly, are believed to increase strength and endurance in the back and improve the function of the lumbar and thoracic back muscles. We'll cover stretching and flexibility routines later that can ease your sore lower back in just a few minutes.

Bone density. Our bones are porous, which is normal. But as we enter middle-age, this porosity can increase, and the bones become less dense, more brittle, and more susceptible to breakage. This condition is called osteoporosis.

Falls are a common cause of bone fractures, but there are others, too, including some that are exercise-induced. Running or jumping on a hard surface, for example, may cause small stress fractures, which are hairline cracks in the bones that can cause pain and lead to larger breaks. The right kinds of exercise, however, can help reverse osteoporosis and make bones stronger:

➢ **High-impact**, weight-bearing exercises include activities like dancing, jumping rope, running and jogging outdoors (with proper athletic shoes to prevent injury), hiking (especially uphill), and playing tennis or racquetball.

➢ **Low-impact**, weight-bearing exercises may be better for those already diagnosed with osteoporosis and include working out on elliptical machines or stair climbers and walking at a brisk moderate pace either outdoors or on a treadmill.

> **Muscle-strengthening** exercises include weightlifting with free weights, like dumbbells and kettle weights, or weight machines with cable-pulled weights, stretching elastic exercise bands, or performing bodyweight calisthenics.

> **Flexibility** exercises can involve stretching (especially after a workout), yoga, and Pilates. Yoga is especially recognized for improving flexibility and balance, which can help prevent falls. If you already have osteoporosis concerns, it's a good idea to check with your doctor or a trained professional physical therapist to make sure you are not straining body parts that are at risk.

Mental health. Exercise reduces symptoms of two of the most common mental and emotional concerns: anxiety and depression. Both of these conditions are frequently caused by stress, which triggers the body's sympathetic response, the well-known "fight or flight" reaction to perceived dangers. The body gets ready for action with elevated heart and breathing rates as well as the release of the energy hormones, adrenaline, and cortisol. In this charged state, anxiety can occur, and when it is continuous over time or chronic, it can lead to autoimmune responses, including chronic inflammation.

> Resistance or cardiovascular exercise takes advantage of the body's state of readiness by effectively putting energy hormones to work and burning the extra glycogen they have sent to your muscles. When the workout is over, and you have cooled down, heart and breathing rates return to normal. The workout also will release beta-endorphin hormones that give you a feeling of elation, and the anxiety can be dissipated.

> ➤ Depression can occur when the parasympathetic response, which cools things down, overdoes it, reducing normal energy levels and depressing the central nervous system. As with anxiety, beta-endorphin hormones can give the person a sense of elation, and the depressive state can be reduced or eliminated.

> ➤ Caveat: Chronic anxiety and depression may not respond sufficiently to exercise, meditation, or yoga, and in those cases, professional care may be necessary.

Dementia. Cognition disorders, especially in people with dementia, may be reduced by exercise. Moreover, those not currently suffering from dementia, and who are physically active regularly with resistance and aerobic exercises, are at reduced risk of developing cognitive impairment and dementia or appreciably slowing its onset.

Cancer. Can the right exercise routines prevent cancer? There is evidence, as the Mayo Clinic reports, that exercise can lower the risk of dying from prostate, breast, and colorectal cancer, and exercise may also help reduce the likelihood of developing other forms of cancer. Exercise may also improve the quality of life and overall fitness for those who have recovered from cancer. Many doctors believe that exercise's role in lowering weight and reducing the likelihood of other diseases keeps the immune system strong, and this helps prevent cancer cells from proliferating, forming tumors, or metastasizing (spreading).

Heart Health

The prevention of heart disease is closely associated with exercise, and with good reason. Exercise can play an important role in preventing heart disease or reducing its risks. Both of the major categories of exercise, resistance and cardiovascular, when performed for sufficient time and with sufficient intensity, can improve overall heart healthiness and contribute to the prevention of heart attacks, heart failure, and strokes.

Heart disease includes atherosclerosis, the build-up of plaque in the coronary arteries that supply the heart with oxygen-rich blood. Over time, as the plaque accumulates, the flow of blood to the heart becomes restricted. Early warnings include angina pectoris, which is a pain in the chest during exercise. Preventing or limiting the build-up of plaque is directly related to controlling the levels of blood lipids.

Can exercise lower blood lipids? The results of studies are encouraging within limits. Blood lipids include HDL (good) cholesterol, which is credited with carrying away LDL (bad) cholesterol, the low density, sponge-like blood lipid which can add to the plaque that clogs arteries, leading to atherosclerosis or coronary heart disease.

Another major blood lipid group is triglycerides, which are fats that circulate in the bloodstream and also can lead to heart disease.

Studies that show exercise-induced reductions of LDL cholesterol and triglycerides and elevated beneficial HDL cholesterol indicate that the **intensity of the exercise is a key factor**. Whether it's weightlifting or aerobics, the workout needs to get the heart rate up and keep it up for at least 25 to 40 minutes three or more times per week.

Controlling hypertension. Exercise can also contribute to lowering hypertension, or high blood pressure, which is a primary cause of strokes.

➤ Exercise and high blood pressure are connected because your heart grows stronger with regular, consistent physical activity. When your heart is stronger, it can pump more blood volume with less exertion. As a result of your heart working less to pump blood, your blood pressure is lowered as the pressure on your arteries is reduced.

➤ Exercise has been clinically proven to lower systolic blood pressure (the first number in your blood pressure reading) by four to nine millimeters of mercury (mm Hg). So, with the right exercise, a systolic pressure of 135 could be lowered to 126, which is within the normal range, and about the same result as from some blood pressure prescription drugs. As a result, for some who have hypertension, regular exercise can reduce or replace a dependency on blood pressure medication.

➤ The benefits of exercise extend to those whose blood pressure is at normal levels, which is less than 130/80 mm Hg. Exercise can help keep your blood pressure from rising as you grow older. Helping you to keep your weight down and maintain a normal BMI is another way exercise helps you to control blood pressure.

Resistance training has also been demonstrated to help protect cardiovascular health. In BMC Public Health (2012), researchers reported that the combination of resistance and aerobic exercise was effective in helping people lose more weight and fat than either of these exercise techniques alone as well as creating increased overall cardiovascular fitness.

➤ The lipid-lowering benefits of resistance training for people with high overall cholesterol were cited in the medical journal Atherosclerosis (2011), showing that those who performed resistance training cleared LDL cholesterol from their bloodstream faster than those who did not train.

High-intensity interval training is generally safe and effective for most people and can take less time. In high-intensity interval training, you alternate exercising at high levels of intensity and exercising at a less intense level for short periods. Even activities such as walking at higher intensities count.

Low-intensity exercise is valuable for helping to lower your weight and to relieve stress, and some studies suggest that even walking at a moderate pace for 150 minutes a week can have positive cardiovascular and overall health benefits. This intensity and duration is an alternative to the frequently recommended 75 minutes per week of intense exercise.

Post-coronary exercise is generally recommended to aid recovery and strengthen the heart, which is a muscle, and like all muscles. benefits from regular exercise. In these cases, the type and intensity of the exercise should be medically supervised.

Now, let's move on to Chapter 2 and see how you can build muscles at age 40, 50, and beyond.

Chapter 2

Build Muscles at 40, 50, and Beyond

Are you skeptical? Do you think that the years have gone by and that you should have gotten into weightlifting and bodybuilding 10 years ago, or even 20 or more years ago? Or you worked out with weights back then, but your career got in the way, and you quit? Those years may be gone, but your opportunity to build those muscles, and gain that strength, is still here, waiting only for you to say to yourself, "This is my chance to make up for lost time and build the body I've always wanted."

Consider when Tug McGraw said, "Ya gotta believe," the admonition that turned around the losing New York Mets, and put them into the 1974 World Series. It's all about positive thinking and having confidence in yourself.

It's not too late. Even if you are middle-aged and have never worked out, even if you're overweight, out of shape, and lack energy, it is not too late for you. This is your time if you have the motivation and commitment to start and continue a weightlifting program. If you are ready, you can fulfill your hopes and dreams of fitness, health, and energy. Yes, you can lift serious weights and build serious lean muscles. You can do this.

The Science of Muscle-Building

To reinforce your confidence and erase any doubts you may have about whether it is possible to become a successful weightlifter at this time in your life, this chapter is going to give you the basics from science and experience to convince you that

371

there are physiological processes that you can initiate that will pay you back generously with results that will surprise you, maybe even astound you.

Science may not be the first thing that comes to mind when planning a muscle-building program, but it is important to ignore the old clichés and anecdotal tales because safely and effectively building lean muscles is based entirely on scientific principles. What does this mean? The scientific method means facts are established by test results that can be consistently repeated and not by opinions and traditions. The principles that apply to young weightlifters also apply to middle-age weightlifters with the understanding that age requires some adjustments to achieve good results safely.

The Concept of Hypertrophy

The muscles we are concerned with are the 650 skeletal muscles that enable us to move and do work. They are made up of muscle fibers which, in turn, are built up from fine thread-like fibers called sarcomeres and myofibrils. These muscle fibers are the fundamental elements of muscular contraction. When you flex a muscle or put it to work, it is within the fibers where the action is taking place. Keep these fibers in mind as we progress because they will be the units of growth that strengthen and build your muscles.

Muscles contract on command when certain nerves, called motor neurons, receive their signals from cells known as the sarcoplasmic reticulum. As your body becomes more conditioned, the signals will become more adept at getting your muscles to contract, and you will become stronger even before muscles are much larger. If you can train to activate your motor neurons effectively, it can jumpstart the processes to build bigger muscles to lift heavier weights. We'll explain this in greater detail in the instructional chapters.

First, do the damage. The process of hypertrophy, the creation of muscle growth, begins with the damage done to muscle fibers during weightlifting. The extreme effort of lifting or pulling heavy weights breaks down some of the muscle fibers that are involved in the hard work; this occurs at the cellular level and is completely normal. Your cells are being sacrificed by doing more work than they are accustomed to.

Next, repair the damage. To repair the damage, the cells use amino acid molecules to fuse into muscle fibers and to form new myofibrils out of strands of protein. This is why protein needs to be an important component of a weightlifter's diet; it is the building block from which the myofibrils are constructed.

Importantly, during this process of hypertrophy:

➤ The myofibrils are not just repaired and rebuilt to their previous size but are made thicker and more numerous. They get slightly larger. They experience growth.

➤ Hypertrophy, or muscle growth, occurs when the production of muscle protein exceeds the previous pre-damage level. On a day-to-day basis, the muscle tissue increments are microscopic, but over time they accumulate, and muscle bulk becomes visible.

Satellite cells. The effectiveness of your hypertrophy is dependent upon what are known as satellite cells, which spur the growth of the myofibrils by increasing muscle protein nuclei and enabling the cells to divide more frequently. According to trainer and coach John Leyva, who is technical editor of the Built

Lean Blog (2020), the degree to which the satellite cells are active is dependent on the type and resistance of the exercises performed and the amount of stress that is placed on the muscles:

1. **Tension of the muscles** is the result of progressively increasing the load that muscles are lifting and pulling, exceeding the amount of resistance they are accustomed to. So if you do bicep curls regularly with 15-pound dumbbells, your biceps and upper arms will retain their current muscle size and strength, but will not grow larger or stronger until you increase the weight to introduce greater resistance and cause stress.

2. **Damage to muscle cells** and tissues releases immune system cells and inflammatory molecules that trigger the activation of satellite cells which, in turn, stimulate the growth of muscle tissue protein and boost hypertrophy. One clear signal that this has occurred is muscle soreness in the hours and even days after your workout. This is due to the damage done during the workout, and it sets the stage for the over-rebuilding of muscle tissue to follow. Much of the soreness is from lactic acid buildup which will dissipate within a day or two.

3. **Metabolic stress** results from intense muscle tension and causes swelling of the cells in and around the muscle. It's the result of the accumulation of blood, which is bringing extra oxygen to the tensed and damaged muscle fibers, plus the arrival of glycogen, the sugar molecules that provide the muscle cells with energy. These effects may contribute to increased rebuilding, but much of the increased muscle size after the workout, while impressive,

is temporary, and the muscles will return to their normal size as the fluids drain from the muscles.

Hormones

The role of hormones in building muscles is frequently debated. This is what is known today about the natural hormones in our bodies:

➢ Testosterone and insulin-like growth factor I (IGH-I) are the two most active hormones that contribute to muscle growth.

➢ While testosterone is at higher levels in men, women also have testosterone (and men also have estrogen), although a woman's testosterone is at a lower level, which is a key reason that men can build muscles more readily than women.

➢ Both men and women can increase strength through weightlifting and other resistance exercises.

While most of our testosterone is not free-roaming or available to affect muscle building, studies show that hard resistance exercise can release more testosterone, which can activate satellite cells, prevent or reduce protein breakdown, increase protein synthesis, and stimulate other anabolic hormones. It may also encourage muscle cell receptors to be more sensitive to free testosterone. Testosterone can also increase the number of neurotransmitters at the site of damaged fiber, help activate tissue growth, and stimulate growth hormone responses.

The bottom line on natural hormones in our bodies is that resistance training can stimulate the release of hormones that further enhance the building of muscle and strength.

Hormones supplements? You are not encouraged to take hormone supplements to build muscle mass unless prescribed by a doctor following a blood test that identifies a hormone deficiency.

Rest and Muscle Loss vs. Muscle Gain

The muscle repairs and rebuilding we've been discussing do not occur during the time while you are actually lifting the weights and damaging the muscle fibers. Instead, muscle growth — hypertrophy — takes place while you, and your muscles, are at rest.

It is during rest that recovery can take place. If the muscles continue to be worked, even to less extreme levels, there will be no opportunity for hypertrophy to do its work and, at best, no repairs can occur. Of greater concern, hard resistance exercise performed too soon after a good weightlifting session can have negative effects:

> ➢ If your muscles do not receive sufficient rest to prepare and conduct their repairs, you can reverse the protein-building process and allow your body to fall into a destructive or catabolic state. Over time, this can lead to muscle loss.

> ➢ The time needed for recovery and hypertrophy after a resistance exercise session is about 24 to 48 hours. So, weightlifting that challenges any specific muscle group should not work that same muscle group for at least one day, preferably two days.

> ➢ If you follow a routine of doing total-body resistance workouts in a single workout session, then you should not have weightlifting or resistance sessions more than three times a week.

Weightlifters over 40. The need for rest and recovery is of special importance to you as a middle-age weightlifter because your recovery time is longer as a function of your age and a slower metabolism. A two-day rest and recovery period after each weightlifting session is ideal for you.

Up the protein. During the rest and recovery days, your diet should be rich in protein since the amino acids that make up protein molecules are needed for the repair of muscle fibers. We'll cover everything you need to know about diet in a later chapter, but for now, assume that you will want to have more meat, fish, dairy, and eggs, all of which are high in complete protein.

Vegetarians and vegans can increase their consumption of beans and other legumes, plus soybeans, buckwheat, and quinoa, which are among the few plant sources of complete protein, including the nine essential amino acids that our bodies need to get from our food.

Over 40: It's Not Too Late

We've just been through the scientific basis for muscle building, and you can appreciate there is no magic or mystery involved. Resistance exercises, followed by adequate rest and recovery and with enough protein in the diet, will build muscles. The cells that compose your muscles get damaged, then repair themselves with added protein, and the cells then over-repair.

As a result, lean muscle tissue increases in size over time, and you grow stronger. Hypertrophy is inevitable if the rules of the game are followed.

Yes, you may be thinking that may work for the young, but you are over 40, or maybe over 50 or 60, and yet now you are being told that it's not too late for you to get those muscles bigger and stronger.

How can this be? With age, your muscles are not as large, some body fat has accumulated, energy isn't the same, and your knees, shoulders, and other joints ache when you bend, crouch, or lift something. Your testosterone level has undoubtedly slipped lower. The porosity of your bones may have increased, maybe osteoporosis is happening, and your bones may be more susceptible to breakage.

An Ideal Time

So, you may ask, all in all, is this really a good time to start, or get back into, serious weightlifting and other forms of resistance exercises? Isn't it too late?

Not only is it not too late, as you have already read, but it's also an ideal time. Stronger, bigger muscles are not a vanity. They are your protection against growing weaker, frail, fragile, less mobile, less flexible, and, here's the big one, less likely to be overweight or obese, and subject to heart disease, diabetes, and a long list of other serious diseases. It's your time right now. You have nothing to lose, and everything — health, longevity, strength, energy and vitality, a great build you can be proud of, self-esteem — to gain.

Weightlifting coach and trainer TC Luomo sums it up in his TC Nation (2019) article by asking if you were an aging professional athlete, presumably having passed age 40, and didn't have what you used to, and you weren't keeping up with the younger athletes, would you give up, retire, and get soft, or would you work harder to regain what you've lost? More to the point, if you wanted to play even better now, even if your joints ache a bit and you're less flexible than before, would you train and work out harder or easier now? His answer is "Harder, of course."

You, at age 40-plus, have unquestionably lost some of the luxuries of your youth so it becomes necessary to train harder — and smarter — to compensate for what the years have taken, gradually and unseen, as a normal part of the aging process. But when you were born, as TC Luomo puts it, you did not have a 40-year expiration date tattooed on your posterior, so what's to stop you from getting back into the muscle-building and fitness game and doing it better than ever before?

New Rules of the Training Game

If training hard and training smart is the formula for success after age 40, there is a set of rules, let's call them guidelines, that will get you where you need to go faster, easier, and more effectively than picking up a barbell, pulling, a cable, stretching a rubber exercise band, or dropping into the plank position and knocking off some push-ups.

The following chapters will guide you through the specific exercises, but these guidelines are meant to give you the big picture, the perspective, on what to do and why to do it.

➢ Quick definition: Reps are repetition, the number of times you lift or pull the weight successively. In total, the repetitions become one set. So an upper-arm workout might be three sets of eight reps of barbell curls, with a one-minute rest between sets.

1. **Breathe deeply**. Unless you have been working hard on the cardiovascular side and have been running, race walking, cycling, swimming, or hitting the elliptical machine or stair climber with sufficient frequency and intensity, you are probably

not close to a high level of aerobic conditioning. OK, you may think, "I get it, for cardiovascular health and to help keep off the pounds, I need to deal with that, but later, because I want to get going with weightlifting first." Yes, the long-term benefits of cardio training are fantastic, but this is about getting you in shape for the immediate term, to ensure that you have the aerobic capacity to breathe and function as you lift weights. This aerobic training will involve three or four days a week when you perform your resistance exercises and will take 10 to 20 minutes starting out. Don't force your heart rate up in the beginning, just be sure that you warm up slowly for two or three minutes. Pick up the pace so that you are breathing hard and deeply for a minute, slow down for one minute, then pick up the pace again and give it a good intensity for one minute, slow again, then fast again. End with a one-minute slowdown.

> ➤ This is an abbreviated version of HIIT, or high-intensity interval training, a compressed form of aerobic conditioning. It will save you the time of slower, dragged out exercise, and has been proven to increase the growth and vibrancy of mitochondria, the energy factories in our muscle cells.

> ➤ Perform this aerobic exercise before you begin the weightlifting, not after. Your objective is to oxygenate your muscle cells before the stress that the resistance exercises create. It is also better to get your heart muscle warmed up slowly rather than forcing it up suddenly with eight reps of lifting a heavy weight.

2.   **Work hard.** Whether you prefer to lift heavy or lighter weights, you are going to be working hard.

You may be lifting heavier weights with fewer reps because some professionals believe it is the best way to catch you up with where you left off, or where you need to start if this is all new to you. That is not to say that you'll be straining, but the recommendations from many trainers are to forget about doing lots of reps with light weights. They say lighter weights with lots of reps may help build endurance but won't address the building of muscle mass or strength.

There is an opposite approach also advocated by some trainers: lifting lighter weights and doing more reps. For example, instead of doing eight to 10 reps with a heavy weight, you lift a lighter weight for 15 to 20 reps. The advantage of lighter weights is that they place less strain on joints, tendons, and ligaments, and since each of us responds uniquely to physical effort and stress, you will need to be the final judge of what works best for you. The following chapters will cover the various exercises and workout routines you can perform.

3.   **Manage the pain.** The expression, "No pain, no gain," became popular in the 1980s when the weightlifting and calisthenics movements began to gain momentum. This expression was subsequently criticized for encouraging people to push past their limits which could lead to injuries ranging from torn ligaments and muscles to joint damage. Today, we know that the responsible approach is to push towards your limits but don't exceed them. Pain is a warning and should not be ignored.

Lifting heavy weights can cause a variety of pains. Joints can creak and ache, muscles can cry out when pushed hard as you try to get that last rep done to conclude a set. These are generally normal but only within limits. Give that last rep a good effort but force it. Do your best but don't punish yourself.

➢ Be especially careful with your shoulders because that set of muscles, called the rotator cuff, is susceptible to tears if subject to shock or excessive stress. Most of your skeletal muscles will hurt too much for you to damage them, and the pain will force you to back off or stop the movement, but your shoulders give little warning when at risk.

4. **Heavy, but not too heavy.** Some weightlifters practice powerlifting, which is very few reps with very heavy weights. This not for you since your 40-plus-year-old joints and connective tissues no longer have the flexibility and resilience they had 20 years ago. So, if you prefer to lift heavy weights, make sure that the weight is not so heavy that you can't do at least eight reps without difficulty. If you can only do three or four reps, the weight is too heavy. Ratchet back until you can find a weight that you max out at eight to 10 reps.

Remember, building muscle and strength takes time and patience. So does losing the extra weight you may be hoping to shed. That's again why the motivation to get started is not enough; you need to commit to going the distance, putting in the months and then making it part of your lifestyle for the years ahead.

5. **Rest, but not too much.** By now, the importance of rest and recovery time has been driven home; you got it, muscles get damaged and need time to build, rebuild, and overbuild. Hypertrophy requires rest. The right amount for the age 40-plus weightlifter is 48 hours. Those two days are what your body needs to get the muscles rebuilt and ready for action. One day of rest might have been enough when you were younger, but at this stage of life, that extra time is needed. If you rush back to the

weights too soon, as you have learned earlier in this chapter, more harm than good can occur.

But there is a limit. Too much rest allows the muscles to get lazy, to forget the conditioning, and start to soften. So two or three days of rest between weightlifting sessions is perfect, four or five days is stretching it a bit, and six or more days rest is too much. Never worry about one missed scheduled workout day, but have the self-discipline to catch up sooner rather than later. Each workout is like an investment, and you want to protect it.

Now, let's head to Chapter 3, which deals with how much weight you should lift.

Chapter 3

How Much You Should Lift

There are two distinctive camps when it comes to the "how much" question: how much weight should a person who is middle-aged be lifting? One side says you should lift heavier weights with fewer reps per set, and the other side advocates taking it easier with the weight and giving the effort more reps. For example, should you lift a 50-pound barbell eight to 10 times to complete one set, or lift a 2-pound barbell 16 to 20 times per set? What about greater extremes, like a 9-pound weight for a maximum of just two reps, or doing 30 to 40 reps with a 12- to 15-pound barbell?

Avoid extremes. For reasons of safety and effectiveness, we can toss out the extremes. As you'll recall from the previous discussion, lifting a weight that you can only raise cleanly and correctly one, two, or at most three times is definitely not recommended for anyone over age 40 whose joints, ligaments, and tendons are no longer as flexible and resilient as when the person was 20 years younger. The other extreme of lifting very light weights for 30 or more times in a set is also not recommended because while it may be safe and not likely to cause injury, the results in building muscle and strength will be minimal.

Between the extremes, there are more moderate alternatives; one that emphasizes building muscle mass and increasing strength, and one which provides benefits of endurance and muscle toning with less risk of injury or strain.

The Heavier Weight Options

The word "heavy" has different meanings to different people and in different situations. A 10pound weight can be considered heavy if you are holding it at arm's length, but light if you are lifting a 10-pound barbell. When it comes to how heavy the weights you lift should be, it's a matter of the desired result, safety, and degrees of intensity.

Moderately Heavy Weights

Advocates of what we'll call the moderately heavier weight approach believe that just because you are a middle-aged weightlifter does not prevent you from lifting heavy weights. If your goal is to develop lean, well-defined muscle mass in the shortest amount of time, moderate heavier weights are the right weights for you. Advocates' experiences lead to the conclusion that the right weight and number of reps per set offer optimal muscle-building results, safely, without over demanding joints and connective tissues.

How heavy? It's easy to determine your safe level of moderately heavier weights at any time in your progress cycle because as you get stronger, the amount you can lift increases in direct proportion to your capacity:

➤ Your capacity is based on the number of reps you can do within a range of weights with eight to 10 reps being the optimal number in a set.

This means you can lift the first six or seven reps without difficulty, but number eight, nine, or at most 10, are barely doable. You should be able to get to this level, but no higher. You will need to make this calculation for each weightlifting exercise:

arms, shoulders, chest, upper body, core and abdominals, back, and legs so that the workout for each muscle group is optimized. If you can only perform five, six, or seven reps, the weight is too heavy, and if you can get past 10 reps, the weight is too light.

You will need to increase the weight level periodically as your strength increases, and when you reach the time when the weight that was tough to raise fully at the eighth to 10th rep is no longer as tough, and you can now do more reps. If the weight can be lifted or pulled more than 10 times, it's time to increase the resistance, not the reps. Be sure that while you are lifting and counting the reps, you are performing the movements by keeping in good form: no jerking, or half-lifts.

Ultra-Heavy vs. Moderately Heavy Weights

You may be wondering about powerlifting. Many seasoned, successful weightlifters believe, unshakably, that for both men and women, the ideal method to build muscle mass is to lift very heavy weights and to increase the weight consistently over time. On the extreme end of this perspective, competitive bodybuilders and powerlifters perform very low reps (from one to three at most) lifting extremely heavy weights, which are 90 percent to 100 percent of the maximum they can lift in one single rep. At the least, bodybuilding and strength optimization is a deep passion for these weightlifters, and to some, it's how they make a living so evidently they do what works.

Why does this ultra-heavy lifting work? Clinical studies in laboratories show that lifting heavier weight, for example, at least 70 percent of a person's maximum one-rep weight activates "fasttwitch type 2 muscle fibers, which play a key role in developing muscle strength and encouraging hypertrophy, which is the process of increasing the size of muscle fiber cells.

But there is a downside. While type 2 muscle fibers may gain more power, they are also subject to early fatigue, and muscle fiber stimulation depends on the duration of how long they are under tension from resistance. If the muscle fibers are not under sufficient tension for enough time, they will be less able to effectively initiate hypertrophy.

Of even greater importance, ultra-heavy weights are not recommended for middle-age weightlifters. It only takes one rep of a very heavy weight to pull or tear a muscle, tendon, or ligament.

This means that for you, at age 40-plus, moderately heavy weights are preferable to ultra-heavy weights:

➤ Because of concerns over ultra-heavy lifting, many aspiring weightlifters are achieving success with the moderately heavy approach: eight to 10 reps at between 70 percent and 75 percent of the maximum you can lift one time. (No need to bring a calculator to the workout; determine the weight you can perform at least eight reps but no more than 10 reps; that is your ideal moderately heavy weight target.)

The Lighter Weight Option

Now let's consider the alternative to lifting heavier weights at the other extreme: many reps with weights (or resistance) you can lift many more times before reaching your maximum effort. We know that lighter weights are less risky since they place less stress on the joints, muscles, tendons, and ligaments. But can lighter weights build the larger, more defined muscles you want and measurably increase your strength?

More is Less

These are the effects when you increase the number of your reps into a higher range, like at least 15 reps per set or even 20 or more. Some who favor lighter weights may lift as many as 32 reps before calling it quits in the set. The specific weight you can manage when doing many reps is estimated to be roughly 50 percent to 60 percent of the maximum you can lift just one time, a single rep. Determination of your ideal lighter weight is similar to moderately heavier weights, but now it's finding out the maximum weight you can lift about 20 to 24 times consecutively.

➤ You may feel like you worked hard after 24 reps, and you have! But the research indicates that you have not lifted a sufficient amount of weight to trigger a type 2, fast twitch response, which is what is needed to promote big muscle growth.

But workouts involving higher reps and lower weights have their own set of benefits because they activate different muscle fibers, called type 1, or "slow-twitch muscle fibers. These responses may not build much muscle and create less power than type 2 responses, but they do increase endurance and are slower to fatigue.

In consequence, a workout with lighter weights and many more reps will not necessarily increase your strength but will build muscular endurance. You will burn more calories with higher reps because these longer workouts help burn fat as well as carbohydrates, thus reducing your total body fat level which can result in a leaner, toned appearance. Your post workout feeling will be more of a glow, and you will be less likely to experience the pain of working out with heavier weights.

Summing up: In considering whether to go for lifting lighter weights and doing more reps or lifting moderately heavy weights with fewer reps, there are positives to each:

➤ With lighter weights and more reps, you will not build muscle or strength compared to lifting moderately heavier weights, but you will increase muscular endurance, and your risk of joint, ligament, tendon, or muscle damage is lower.

➤ Lifting moderately heavy weights will get you to your muscle-building and strength increasing goals, but be aware there is a higher risk of strain or injury. Be careful not to overdo the weights, and let the number of reps be your guide. If you can't lift the weight eight times, it's too heavy.

Middle-Age Celebrity Weightlifters

Becoming a weightlifter after age 40, or returning to weightlifting at this age after a long hiatus, is not something new or unique. On the contrary, men and women who do not want to accept the negative consequences of maturity, who want to slow the aging process and maintain good health, are working out with weights in health clubs, fitness centers, gyms, and at home. Their routines may vary from individual to individual, but they are united in the common goals of wanting to be stronger, and to look stronger.

Middle-agers working out and increasing their musculature, getting stronger, and shaping up is going on all around us, and a visit to a fitness center will confirm that it's not just younger people but many of us of all ages who are curling dumbbells, lifting barbells, swinging kettle weights, pulling cables, stretching exercise bands, and doing pull-ups. The treadmills, ellipticals, and cycles are frequently occupied by older men and women who are including a good cardiovascular workout in their routines.

To give you other examples of middle-age weightlifting and physical fitness advocates, we can turn to some action-hero celebrities for inspiration: Jason Statham, Daniel Craig, Dwayne "The Rock" Johnson, and Hugh Jackman.

Jason Statham

Jason Statham's films include The Mechanic, Furious 7, Death Race, and Hobbs and Shaw. In these and many other films and shows, we know him as an action hero scaling buildings, overcoming adversaries, and being an all-around tough guy. But Jason is no kid, and at age 52, he's working out most days of the week as hard as he ever has, reminiscent of his younger days when he was a diver and footballer. That is why he maintains an enviable physique and looks and feels like his younger self.

What's his routine? Jason's objectives are to preserve lean muscle, get rid of any extra body fat, and stay strong and flexible. He wants to keep his metabolism from slowing down, and he attributes his fitness to his diet as much as his workouts. We'll cover diet in a later chapter, but here are the highlights of what he eats.

A responsible diet. Jason follows what appears to be close to the Mediterranean diet, which focuses on oats and other whole grains, nuts and seeds, cold-water fish (high in omega 3 antioxidants), lean chicken, brown rice, lots of fresh fruit, and a variety of vegetables. Protein is a priority to keep building muscle. He believes that about 95 percent of his diet is healthy, though he allows himself some chocolate (dark chocolate is now recognized as beneficial, so no guilt needed). To his credit and nutritional advantage, he avoids greasy fried foods (as everyone concerned about their health should do).

You will see a full day of Jason's nutritional selections in Chapter 6, but here are the highlights to give you the idea of what makes a great diet for a middle-age athlete who wants to get stronger, stay fit, and keep healthy:

➤ **Breakfast** begins with fresh fruits, including strawberries and pineapple, followed by oatmeal, which is loaded with cholesterol-reducing fiber, then a good protein hit with poached eggs.

➤ **Lunch** often includes brown rice, which provides quality carbohydrates, fiber, vitamins, minerals, and some protein. Jason adds steamed vegetables for added nutrition; this combination is actually a vegan lunch which he thinks is good on occasion. He often adds a bowl of hot miso soup, which Jason thinks is delicious and healthy (it is but be aware of the sodium level if you're concerned about hypertension).

➤ **Snack** time is nut time in the form of the cashews, almonds, and walnuts he likes to crunch on. Nuts also come into play with peanut butter, but not the processed, sugar loaded commercial brands. Jason stays with the unprocessed, all-natural version which is ground peanuts and nothing else. (Again, a head's up on salt; salt-free is better for you.

➤ **Dinner** is the heavier protein meal with lean beef one night, chicken or fish on another. Salmon or other cold-water fish are the healthiest for you, and try to keep the chicken lean. Jason's evening meal includes both vegetables and a leafy green salad. (Hint: Start the evening meal with a large green salad, and you'll eat less of the higher calorie foods to follow.)

An awesome workout. Here's one day of a seven-day workout that Jason performs. This is his workout, not yours, so be inspired to work towards it someday. More practically, say to yourself that if he can do all that powerlifting, what you will be learning in the following chapter is pretty easy by comparison. Remember, Jason Statham has been working out with increasing intensity all life, so don't feel you're not measuring up. If Jason was just starting on his exercise program at middle-age or getting back to weightlifting after a 15- or 20-year hiatus, he'd probably be following the same program you'll be following. Here's his actual Day 1:

Deadlift One-Rep Max Progression

This involves a series of warm-ups and one-rep bench press exercises, paving the way for a solitary goal: the almighty deadlift (i.e., a one-repetition max of the heaviest weight you can lift at one time).

As a warm-up to get the blood circulating and oxygenate the muscles, Jason first hops on the rowing machine and rows for 10 minutes at a moderate pace. Then, a pyramid circuit in which he does one rep of each of these three: barbell squat, press-up (same as push-up), and ring pull-ups using a light weight and his bodyweight. One round of the circuit is done, then repeated but with two reps; pause, again each one for three reps, then four, then five reps. Then he descends the circuit with four reps, three, two, and finally one rep.

So now Jason is warmed up and ready to go to work. If you feel exhausted just reading about his warm-up, fasten your seatbelt for what's about to follow.

Jason Statham's deadlift workout is the ultra-heavy weightlifting we discussed in the previous section, and it was agreed it is not for you. But Jason has his agenda, and here it is. A deadlift is the buzzword for the one-rep maximum weight routine. You will see he starts heavy, gets heavier, then gets really heavy, maxing out at 365 pounds. Here is Jason's deadlift sequence for the barbell squat:

1. 10 reps lifting 135 pounds, followed by one-minute rest.
2. 5 reps lifting 185 pounds, followed by two-minute rest.
3. 3 reps lifting 235 pounds, followed by three-minute rest.
4. 2 reps lifting 285 pounds, followed by three-minute rest.
5. 1 rep lifting 325 pounds, followed by three-minute rest.
6. 6. 1 rep lifting 350 pounds, followed by three-minute rest.
7. 1 rep lifting 360 pounds, followed by three-minute rest.
8. 1 rep lifting 365 pounds, followed by three-minute rest, then cool down.

Cool down for Jason is doing footwork on a trampoline for 10 minutes; an alternative could be 10 to 15 minutes on a treadmill at low speed and elevation.

While the amount of weight being lifted is impressive, notice the way the weights are increased gradually and that rest between lifts increases as the weights increase. Yes, the final weight is extremely heavy, but Jason worked up to it gradually with adequate rest between lifts.

Day 2 involves five different exercises, which are less on weights and more on reps, done in sequence, and which Jason calls the Big Five 55 Workout. He alternates between five exercises: front squats, pull-ups, push-ups, power clean lifts (bend down, lift the barbell to the chest, hold erect, then lower), and hanging on the pull-up bar while pulling knees up to elbows.

He does 10 sets, with minimal rest in between that eventually total 55 reps for each of the five exercises.

Statham alternates between the five exercises and performs the entire circuit 10 times. He starts with 10 reps, then goes down to nine, then eight, and so on, making for a total of 55 reps per exercise. There should be minimal rest time between each set.

Day 3, for a change of pace, is mostly aerobic done entirely on the rowing machine. He warms up slowly on the machine for 10 minutes, then performs six high-intensity sprints, each covering 500 meters, in one minute, 40 seconds average time, which is very fast. He cools down by walking 500 meters carrying two heavy kettle weights.

Daniel Craig

The most rugged and muscular of the actors to star in the James Bond movies, Daniel Craig looks like he can handle any situation or antagonist. His workouts have built a physique that looks powerful, yet functional, with flexibility and speed as well as considerable strength. What is his workout like?

He starts the week performing a power circuit that works the full body, not just one or two muscle groups, and performs three sets of 10 reps. This series includes exercises for the arms and shoulders, chest, abdominals and center body core, upper and lower back, and the legs, including glutes, quadriceps, hamstrings, and calves. For the next four days, Daniel exercises limited muscle groups, performing four sets of 10 reps. Every session concludes with a five-minute sprints interval on the treadmill or outside the fitness center. His trainer then has him take off from the gym for the weekend, but he has Daniel do some light yoga-style stretching and easy aerobic exercises, usually a swim or a run at a slow or moderate pace.

Day 2 workout. For example, the muscle group that Daniel exercises on Day 2 works the chest, shoulders, and back. The workout includes these four exercises, which you can try because they involve moderately heavy weights performed for 10 reps each:

1. Incline barbell bench press. The starting position is lying back on a bench raised to an incline. The barbell is raised to shoulder height with the palms facing forward. Exhale fully and press up the barbell with both arms. Hold in the fully extended position, then inhale before slowly returning to the starting position. Daniel performs four sets of 10 reps, with 90-second rests between sets.

2. Pull-ups are a bodyweight calisthenic exercise and begin by reaching up to grasp the pull-up bar or handles with palms facing forward and hands about shoulder-width apart. Slowly pull up to bring the chin to the level of the bar or handles, then slowly lower fully to the starting position. Squeeze your shoulder blades as you lift and exhale. Inhale as you lower back down. Again, perform four sets of 10 reps, with 90-second rests between sets.

3. Incline press-ups are a modified version of the classic push-up, and they are a little easier since you are not lowering all the way down and lifting up from the floor position. Place your hands shoulder-width apart on a bench and extend your legs fully to the rear. You should be up on your toes. Begin with your arms fully extended and slowly lower your chest to the bench, exhaling as you descend. Pause momentarily, and then raise fully back up

to the starting position, inhaling as you rise. Perform four sets of 10 reps with 90-second rests between sets.

4. Dumbbell incline fly begins by lying on an incline bench and holding a dumbbell in each hand. Begin with arms fully extended upward. Slowly lower your arms outwards to the side until your arms are parallel to the floor or as far as you can comfortably lower without pain. It may be easier to have a slight bend at the elbow. Bring your arms up above you again, then repeat the movement. As with the other exercises in this group, perform four sets of 10 reps with 90- second rests between sets.

On other days, Daniel Craig performs a series of leg-strengthening exercises, and bicep curls and dips for arms and shoulders. Then, the weekend and no weights, but then on Monday, it's back to the full-body workout after the two days of rest.

Dwayne "The Rock" Johnson

The Rock needs no introduction, having gone from college athlete to WWE sensation to action movie star. Unlike many other Hollywood stars who are well built, Dwayne may be the best-built, most muscular star ever with the possible exception of Arnold Schwarzenegger. Dwayne makes it clear he worked hard to get where he is and to achieve his huge muscles, but he is always open to share his experience and practices to benefit others. While it is doubtful that any of us aspire to build up the muscle bulk he showed us in Fast Five or Hercules or to be anywhere near Dwayne's level, there may be value in letting him share his advice. He is inspiring, there's no doubt of that.

He starts with cardio. First thing in the morning every morning, The Rock hits the elliptical cross-training machine for 30 to 50 minutes of hard aerobics.

Then breakfast. He begins his day's fueling with a protein-intense breakfast. For example, on most days he consumes five serious meals, and the first one, after the early cardio and a shower, includes no less than:

➢ Two cups of cooked oatmeal (starts with one cup of dry oats)
➢ Three egg whites plus one whole egg (egg whites are almost pure protein)
➢ 10-ounce steak or other lean meat (for extra protein)
➢ One glass watermelon juice

The remaining four or so meals of the day each include an eight-ounce serving of either fish, chicken, or beef, along with vegetables. like broccoli, asparagus, and potato, plus lots of eggs and egg whites. The last meal is limited to 10 egg whites and casein protein.

The workout begins later in the morning. The Rock makes it as tough and as intense as he can to follow his philosophy of "epic pain, epic gain." This is not a workout discipline that you will want to emulate, but what Dwayne goes through to achieve his massive muscles and sharp definition gives you an idea of what the human body is capable of building. A small fraction of these muscles can still be impressive.

He works out six days a week and varies the routine from day to day to rest different muscle groups and for variety to prevent boredom.

Day 1 focuses on the legs. Note the moderate to high level of reps.	**Day 2** is devoted to back and shoulder muscles.
Barbell Squat: 4 sets of 12 reps	Pull-Ups: 3 sets to failure
Thigh Abductor: 4 sets of 12 reps	Bent-Over Barbell Row: 4 sets of 12 reps
Hack Squat: 4 sets of 12 reps	Wide-Grip Lat Pulldown: 4 sets of 12 reps
Leg Press: 4 sets of 25 reps	Bent-Over Barbell Row: 4 sets of 12 reps
Leg Extensions: 3 sets of 20 reps	One-Arm Dumbbell Row: 4 sets of 12 reps
Single-Leg Hack Squat: 4 sets of 12 reps	Barbell Deadlift: 3 sets of 10 reps
Romanian Deadlift: 4 sets of 10 reps	Inverted Row: 3 sets, to failure
Barbell Walking Lunge: 4 sets of 25 reps	Dumbbell Shrug: 4 sets of 12 reps
Seated Leg Curl: 3 sets of 20 reps	Back Hyperextensions: 4 sets of 12 reps

The week continues with Day 3 for the shoulders, Day 4 for arms and abs, Day 5 for the legs again, and Day 6 for the chest. Day 7 is a rest day with no workouts, and The Rock is reported to indulge in ice cream on this one day a week. Well deserved, it seems.

Hugh Jackman

During the 17 years he played Wolverine, a mutant with the steel knife-blade hands, in the X Men movies, Hugh Jackman has been bulking up well-defined muscles by following a tough workout routine and a high-protein diet. His career has extended beyond action hero to a lead role in the musical Les Miserable.

A balanced diet. Yes, extra protein has been an essential part of Hugh's diet, but he is not a protein-obsessed fanatic. He balances his diet with healthy, unprocessed carbohydrates, including vegetables like sweet potatoes, broccoli, spinach, and avocado, which is credited with omega-3 antioxidants, plus niacin, beta-carotene, riboflavin, folate, magnesium, potassium, pantothenic acid, and vitamins. Carbs plus protein also come from whole grains, notably oatmeal and brown rice, which are high in antioxidants, vitamins, minerals, and digestion benefiting fiber. Oats are also believed to lower LDL (bad) cholesterol.

Protein sources include eggs, fish for omega-3 fats, chicken, and lean beef. All in all, it's a protein-rich version of the Mediterranean diet, although there's no indication, he also includes nuts, seeds, and beans in his diet.

Bulk and cut muscle. Hugh's trainer introduced him to a dual strategy workout routine with one type focusing on building muscle mass and the other aiming to provide more definition. Low-intensity/high-intensity intervals were included to emphasize lean muscle and minimize body fat.

Hugh's training has followed progressive overload, which is gradually increasing the weight being pulled, pushed, and lifted during each workout to ensure continual increases in strength. During a four-week cycle, the weight was increased for each of the first three weeks, then reduced for the fourth week with a corresponding increase in the number of reps.

The exercises that Hugh performed included barbell bench press, back squat, weighted pullup, and barbell deadlift, according to this four-week plan with progressions during the first three weeks:

Hugh Jackman's four-week progressive overload schedule:

Week 1:	Week 2:
5 reps at 60% of maximum in set one	4 reps at 65% of maximum in set one
5 reps at 65% of maximum in set two	4 reps at 75% of maximum in set two
5 reps at 70% of maximum in set three	4 reps at 85% of maximum in set three
5 reps at 75% of maximum in set four	4 reps at 85% of maximum in set four
Week 3:	**Week 4:**
3 reps at 70% of maximum in set one	10 reps at 40% of maximum in set one
3 reps at 80% of maximum in set two	10 reps at 50% of maximum in set two
3 reps at 90% of maximum in set three	10 reps at 60% of maximum in set three
3 reps at 90% of maximum in set four	10 reps at 90% of maximum in set four

Interestingly, Hugh's trainer concentrated his workout with only five major exercises to build arms and shoulders, chest, abs, back, and legs.

Now, with your motivation to build muscles and begin a successful weightlifting and fitness program, it's time to move on to your action plan in Chapter 4.

Chapter 4

Optimal Exercise Routines and Recovery Practices

With the lessons and insights, we've now covered, and with an understanding of why heavy weights have the advantage over lighter weights, you are ready to develop your own exercise selection and recovery routine. This chapter is where you will learn the exercise routines that you can select to develop a personalized, effective schedule of workouts. While you will be doing many of your exercises with heavy weights, they may not be as heavy as the weights you lifted when you were younger (if you ever lifted weights during that time of your life) or that you may see others lifting.

Weightlifting is not limited to iron weights and machines with cables. It also includes bodyweight calisthenics, movements that require only the weight of your body to provide the necessary resistance for tough workouts that lead to impressive results.

To supplement calisthenics, those working out at home without equipment can purchase stretch bands or tubes that can be used to replicate many of the exercises performed at fitness centers with weights and progressive resistance machines. The exercises presented in this chapter will be weightlifting with weights and bodyweight calisthenics.

Most weightlifting exercises can be performed without risk at age 40-plus as long as you work progressively and don't try to lift too much. Stay fully aware of the necessary recovery time after weightlifting to let hypertrophy, the rebuilding and growth process, function and be cognizant that after age 40, hypertrophy takes longer and the risk of injury from overwork is greater. As you were advised in this book's introduction, patience will be rewarded with results; it takes time as well as effort to build lean, well-defined muscles.

The Right Routine for Your Age

Your age, like most numerical designations, is relative. At age 40, or 50, or 60, your ability to perform a range of weightlifting exercises with varying weights and reps depends on your current physical state.

Your condition is based on a diversity of factors, including how aging has affected you, like the degrees of joint and tendon flexibility, and how they may have stiffened; how your health is; whether your muscles have atrophied from lack of use; and whether your cardiovascular system is running at full functionality. As it has been said, "It's not the years, it's the miles," meaning your condition is not just about age, but what damage has occurred from under-use or over-use. It is important to treat your body with respect for its actual condition and not what you hope or wish it to be. Realism is important if you are to achieve your expectations of greater strength, bigger muscles, and overall fitness.

First, Do No Harm

Yes, you will be working hard and challenging your muscles, joints, tendons, and ligaments, but your objective is to build and grow, not to punish and injure.

Whatever your condition now, respect your body as being middle-aged and follow the Hippocratic doctrine of "first, do no harm." You may have the best of intentions, but if you start out doing exercises that are best left to experienced, well-conditioned athletes or try to lift more weight than your joints or ligaments can handle, you are taking several unnecessary risks:

> **Injury** from a torn shoulder rotator cuff to a strained muscle that holds your kneecap in place. These kinds of injuries can take months to heal. There is minimal risk of injury if you work within your zone of ability.

> **Overuse**, meaning the muscles have been overextended, and the damage done to the fibers and cells will not repair and recover during the normal two days of rest. As a result, muscles will not grow and may atrophy, or get smaller.

> **Pain**, since lifting or pulling too much weight or doing too many reps can hurt and could end up diminishing your enthusiasm and motivation for strength training. Always consider pain to be a warning.

Your age, physical condition, health, and other factors make you unique. This is why you are being counseled to pay no attention to other weightlifters. They have their limits, and you have yours. There is no value in over-lifting, in pushing or pulling too much early in your middle age return to weightlifting, only to injure yourself with a strained or torn muscle and shut down what you have just started.

Exercises to Avoid in Middle-Age

Aside from lifting too much weight, there are popular exercises you may be familiar with and plan to include in your routine, but experts advise you to let these go and avoid the risks of injury. Tell yourself that you have outgrown these exercises and leave them to the youngsters:

> **Overhead press**. Standing and raising a barbell above your head and lowering to your shoulders behind your head puts excess pressure on your shoulders, neck, and spine.

> **Bench press**. Lying on a bench and pushing a heavy barbell upwards may be good for your chest at age 25, but at 45, an excess strain is put on your pectoral (chest) muscles, wrists, and shoulders.

> **Crunches**. These slight lifts of the head and shoulders while on your back replaced the sit-up as safer, but at middle age, crunches put too much pressure on your neck and spine. Avoid pinched nerves and work your abs with less risk by doing leg raises, hanging leg raises, and planks.

> **Deadlifts**. Bending down and lifting a barbell to your chest is dangerous to your back. As a minimum, deadlifts can cause chronic back pain and may result in more serious back injuries.

> **Leg presses**. Sitting and pushing a heavy weight with your legs bent seems innocent enough, but the pressure on middle-aged hips and knees can lead to joint pain. Instead, strengthen your legs with low-impact lunges while carrying a moderate weight dumbbell or no added weight.

> **Lateral pull-downs**. You sit on a bench, facing the machine, reach up and pull-down a bar to your chest, or worse, behind your neck. At middle-age, this maneuver risks pinched neck nerves and torn rotator-cuff shoulder muscles.

Also, while you are encouraged to include cardiovascular training into your workouts, be aware that running on hard surfaces can cause permanent knee damage, and you should consider limiting running to a treadmill or on grass if you want to run outdoors. Runners need to wear quality shoes designed for cushioned landing and to help prevent pronation, or outward foot rotation.

Equipment You Will Need (and Alternatives)

Fitness centers. The practice of strength training requires forms of resistance that are the basis of building lean, defined muscle, and making you stronger. There is usually a full range of weightlifting equipment found in a health club or fitness center, such as free weights like dumbbells, barbells, and kettlebells, plus progressive exercise machines with cables and weights that you can pull or push to work different muscle groups. A well-equipped fitness center or gym will also have rubber stretch tubes, adjustable benches, and a pull-up bar. These fitness centers generally require monthly membership fees unless you live in an apartment building or residential community that provides a fitness center as an amenity.

Home gym. A good alternative to a health club membership is to create your own small home gym, which could include a selection of free weights, a portable pull-up and chin-up bar, and a selection of stretchable rubber bands or tubes. The small investment in this equipment may be quickly amortized by the savings in fitness center monthly membership fees.

Bodyweight calisthenics. An even less costly way to build muscles and strength is to use your own weight as the resistance. Examples include familiar push-ups, pull-ups and chin-ups, leg raises, planks, and dips. There are many other calisthenics movements that can round out a full, total-body workout.

Group 1 of weightlifting exercises is based on having access to weights and other resistance equipment. Group 2, calisthenics, is almost all equipment-free and can be performed at home. You are encouraged to try exercises from both groups to add variety to your workouts and give a wider range of challenges to your muscles.

Each exercise has images of the movement and a link to a YouTube video demonstration so you can learn the movements correctly.

➤ Skip Ad. Many of the videos will begin with a short commercial, but after five seconds a "Skip Ad" box will appear on the lower right corner of the screen, and a quick click will get the exercise demo going.

Group 1: Weightlifting Exercises

The following weightlifting exercises have been selected to provide good strength and muscle building results with a low risk of injury. Select exercises to work specific muscle groups, and then vary them so you have at least one, preferably two, rest days before working the same muscle groups.

- ➤ **Tip:** Breathe out as you lift, and inhale as the weights are lowered.
- ➤ **Tip:** The weight you select should be what you can lift eight to 10 reps, and you should perform three sets with 60 to 90 seconds rest between sets.

1. Dumbbell Incline Press

You will develop your chest, upper arms, shoulders, and lats (sides of the upper chest) with the dumbbell incline press.

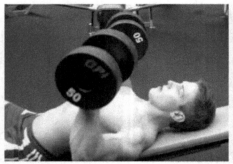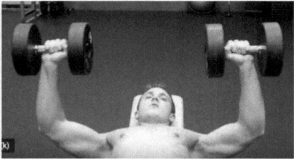

Fig 1. Dumbbell Incline Press

Tip: Use a lighter weight than you think appropriate when you perform the dumbbell incline press for the first few times. You do not want to over-lift or be trying to control the dumbbells because they are too heavy.

Tip: If the dumbbells are still hard to control, try the movement with a barbell. Use a wide grip (just past shoulder width) to simulate the movement with barbells.

Link to demonstration video: "How to: dumbbell incline chest press." YouTube.

https://www.youtube.com/watch?v=8iPEnn-ltC8

2. Seated Cable Rows

This is a compound exercise that builds up the shoulders, abdominals, and core, both front and back.

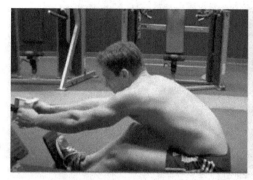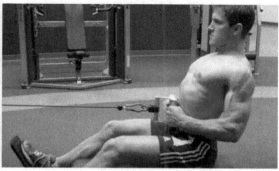

Fig 2. Seated Cable Rows

Tip: This is an excellent exercise for the hard-to-reach back muscles, but be careful to pull a weight you can manage without straining your back.

Tip: As you reach the full extend of the pull-back, squeeze your shoulder blades together for additional conditioning.

Link to demonstration video: "How to: seated low row." YouTube.

https://www.youtube.com/watch?v=GZbfZ033f74

3. Dumbbell Split Squats

This leg exercise specifically works the quadriceps, the major muscles at the front of your thighs.

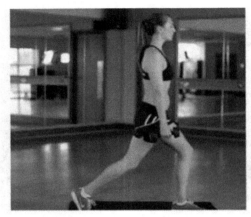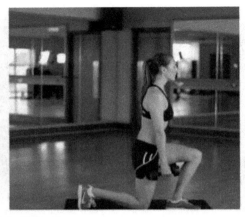

Fig 3. Dumbbell Split Squats

Tip: Do not lean backward to maintain balance and keep control of the movement, but a slight forward lean is OK.

Tip: Perform eight to 10 repetitions with the same leg forward, then switch to the other leg, and repeat to complete one set, remembering to keep your weight on the lead foot.

Tip: If you find doing eight reps with each leg too difficult, use lighter dumbbells and few reps for the first week; do three sets with a rest of 90 seconds between sets.

Link to demonstration video: "Dumbbell split squat - fitness gym training." YouTube.

https://www.youtube.com/watch?v=MEG6blZtUpc

4. Bent-Over Rows with Dumbbells

This will isolate the muscles in your back, especially the rhomboids, lats, and trapezoids. Secondarily you will be working the upper arm biceps and posterior deltoids, and you will also help stabilize your core and lower body.

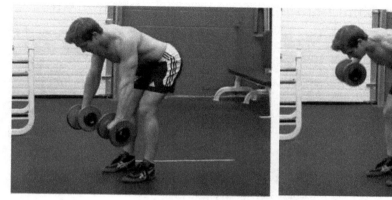

Fig. 4. Bent Over Rows with Dumbbells

Tip: If you feel your back straining, reduce the amount of the forward bend, which will take some pressure off your spine.

Tip: An alternative grip is to hold the dumbbells with your palms facing to the rear. (You can alternate grip with palms to sides and palms to rear between reps or sets; this will increase the muscles involved.)

Link to demonstration video: "How to: dumbbell bent-over row." YouTube.

https://www.youtube.com/watch?v=6TSP1TRMUzs

5. Dumbbell Upright Row

This is a good shoulder-strengthening exercise and has considerable benefits when performed correctly. However, trainers caution that if performed incorrectly, upright rows can do more harm than good, so pay close attention to your form. Start with lighter weights to play it safe when starting out.

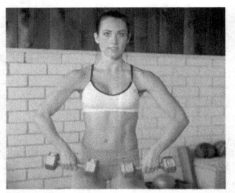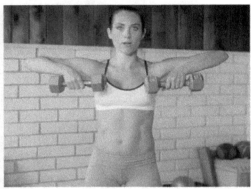

Fig 5. Dumbbell Upright Row

Tip: Since you will be starting with lighter weights for safety, perform 12 to 14 reps for each of three sets with 60 seconds rest between sets. If you can't do 12 reps, reduce the weight you are lifting.

Link to demonstration video: "How to upright row - proper form and tips." YouTube.

https://www.youtube.com/watch?v=VIoihl5ZZzM

6. *Standing Barbell Curl*

This is an exercise that weightlifters favor to build their upper arms, notably the biceps. It may also be performed with two dumbbells, but a barbell is preferred when starting out because it's easier to control and will tend to follow the correct path of up-and-down movements.

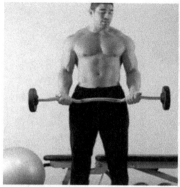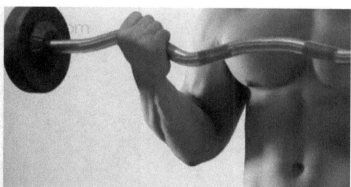

Fig 6. Standing Barbell Curl

Tip: Be careful to control the bar, lifting it with both of your arms doing equal work (which will keep the bar parallel to the floor), and do not jerk the weight upwards, or let it drop down too fast. As with all weightlifting, slower is better.

Tip: If you are able, perform three sets of eight to 10 reps with a rest of 60 to 90 seconds between sets. If you find doing eight reps too difficult, use a lighter barbell.

Link to demonstration video: "How to do a barbell curl | arm workout." Howcast/YouTube.

https://www.youtube.com/watch?v=kwG2ipFRgfo

7. Dumbbell Side Lateral Raises

These side raises are excellent for building your shoulders and giving you a wide upper body. It challenges your rear deltoids and trapezius, but it's important to perform the movements correctly because, as you know by now, the rotator cuff muscles in your shoulder can be susceptible to strains and tears.

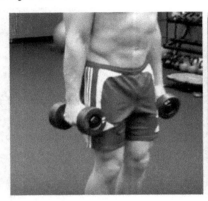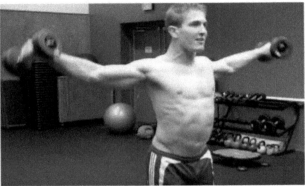

Fig 7. Dumbbell Side Lateral Raises

Tip: If you feel pain, especially as you reach the top of the movement, stop and lower the weight. Be careful not to go any higher in the following reps (your range of motion should increase over time).

Tip: Perform three sets of eight to 10 reps, with a rest of 60 to 75 seconds between sets. If you can't make it to eight reps in the first set, stop when you must, then reduce the weight for the next two sets.

Link to demonstration video: "How to: dumbbell lateral side raise." YouTube.

https://www.youtube.com/watch?v=3VcKaXpzqRo

Group 2: Calisthenic Exercises

Bodyweight calisthenics can be performed at home, or anywhere, with little or no special equipment, and they should be part of your weightlifting program even if you have access to a fitness center's equipment. You may combine weightlifting and calisthenics in a single workout or on alternate days. Just be sure to avoid working the same muscle groups on consecutive days.

Tip: For all exercises performed on the floor, use a yoga, exercise mat, or carpeting for cushioning. It's important to protect your spine.

Tip: Breathe out as you lift or push yourself up, and inhale as your bodyweight is lowered.

Tip: You can't vary your bodyweight, so for optimal effects, slow down the pace of the movements so you can lift or pull about 10 reps. For example, if you are finding it hard to do 10 push-ups, take a few seconds longer during each up and down.

Tip: Perform three sets with 60 to 75 seconds rest between sets.

8. Planks

The plank looks simple enough, just holding a position, but it is a static stability exercise credited as outstanding for strengthening the core, which includes your abdominals, back, and sides. The plank is recommended as a replacement for sit-ups, which may cause spinal damage through disc compression.

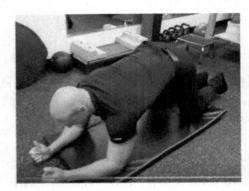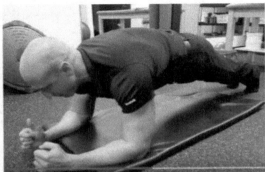

Fig 8. Planks

Tip: Correct posture is critical. The objective is to keep your back straight, not sagging or with your buttocks pushing upward. Do not raise your head, but hold it so you are looking at the floor.

Tip: This is the plank position, or pose, and it is held for 10 seconds up to one minute. One plank rep is considered one set, so you should perform three planks with a 60- to 90-second rest between planks.

Tip: Within several weeks, you should be able to hold your plank, with a straight back, for 45 to 60 seconds.

Link to demonstration video: "How to do a proper plank." Body Mind Wellness Clinic/YouTube.

https://www.youtube.com/watch?v=gvHVdNVBu6s

9. Bodyweight Squats

This is a classic bodyweight exercise that is an excellent builder for the quadriceps and hip flexors.

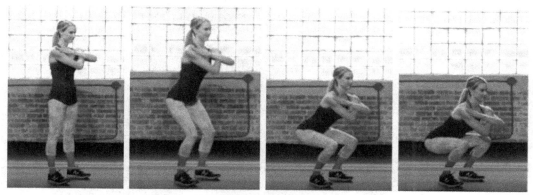

Fig 9. Bodyweight Squats

Tip: If you find doing eight reps too difficult, perform fewer reps for the first week or two until your legs are accustomed to the movement.

Tip: If your knees hurt during, or following, the squats, limit your descent to just before your thighs are parallel with the floor, but not past the point when the knee pain begins.

Link to demonstration video: "How to do a body-weight squat." Health Magazine/YouTube.

https://www.youtube.com/watch?v=LyidZ42Iy9Q

10. Lying Leg Raises

Leg raises, like the plank, can replace sit-ups and crunches (partial sit-ups) to work the abdominals and core. This movement also stretches the hip flexors, hamstrings, and glutes.

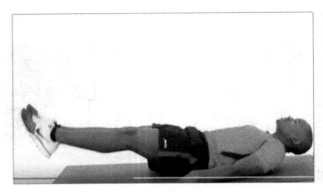 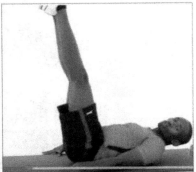

Fig 10. Lying Leg Raises

Tip: You may find it easier to raise your legs if you slide your hands under your hips; alternatively, place a folded towel under your hips. This may also prevent straining your lower back muscles.

Link to demonstration video: "How to do lying leg raises for abs." YouTube.

https://www.youtube.com/watch?v=UvcTNVbjTYo

11. Push-Ups

This is a classic bodyweight exercise that has stood the test of time, being safe to perform, and returning good results in strengthening many muscle groups, including arms, shoulders, back, abdominals, and core.

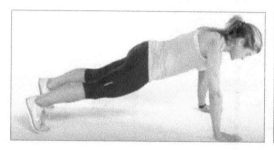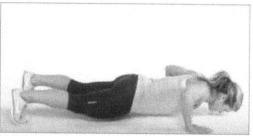

Fig 11. Push Ups

Tip: As you get stronger, and push-ups get easier, slow down each cycle, taking longer to go down and back up. This can challenge your muscles more than simply increasing the reps.

Tip: If you are having trouble doing even one or two push-ups, begin by keeping your weight on your knees instead of your toes. Or, place your hands on a bench, so you are not fully lowering to the floor.

Link to demonstration video: "How to do a push-up." Dr. Oz/YouTube.

https://www.youtube.com/watch?v=rjc0O7OXS3g

12. Pull-Ups and Chin-Ups

Pull-ups and chin-ups will build your upper back, shoulders, and core; chin-ups also give your biceps good resistance. You may have done pull-ups in high school, and if you thought they were tough then, wait until you try them now at middle-age. But you can work your way back and get quite good at pull-ups.

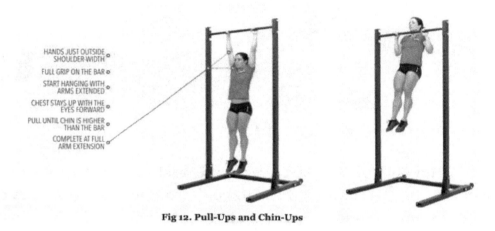

HANDS JUST OUTSIDE SHOULDER-WIDTH

FULL GRIP ON THE BAR

START HANGING WITH ARMS EXTENDED

CHEST STAYS UP WITH THE EYES FORWARD

PULL UNTIL CHIN IS HIGHER THAN THE BAR

COMPLETE AT FULL ARM EXTENSION

Fig 12. Pull-Ups and Chin-Ups

Tip: You may alternate pull-ups and chin-ups. For example, set one, pull-ups; set two, chin-ups; and set three, return to pull-ups. The only difference is the grip (palms forward, wide grip for pull-ups; palms back, narrow grip for chin-ups).

Tip: Repeat the cycle until you have performed five to eight reps. If you can only do one or two reps, that's OK; it's better to do fewer pull-ups in the correct form than to do more by lifting partially, or going too fast.)

Link to demonstration video: "The strict pull-up and chin-up." YouTube.

https://www.youtube.com/watch?v=HRV5YKKaeVw

13. Hanging Leg Lifts

This exercise is another good challenge to the core muscles, especially your abdominals, back, and shoulders. It requires a pull-up bar and can be approached in three gradual stages. You are free to go directly to Stage 3, but it's a good idea to make sure you can perform Stages 1 and 2 before trying Stage 3.

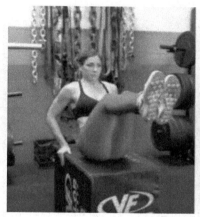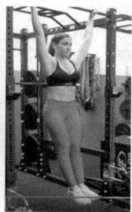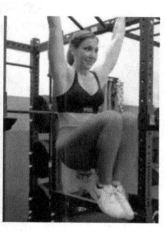

Fig 13. Hanging Leg Lifts

Tip: In the early stages of your fitness program, you may find hanging from the bar difficult. In time you will get stronger, but if necessary, practice the first two stages (as shown in the video demo).

Tip: In the interim, before you can perform this exercise, rely on lying leg raises and planks to tighten your core muscles.

Link to demonstration video: "Hanging leg raises done right." YouTube.

https://www.youtube.com/watch?v=lS5B0MmLgZs

14. Triceps Bench Dips

This simple exercise can be performed using a bench, low table, or chair, and it is one of the best movements to isolate and work the triceps muscles at the rear of your upper arms. If you use a chair, make sure it is solid and will not tip forward as you place your weight on it.

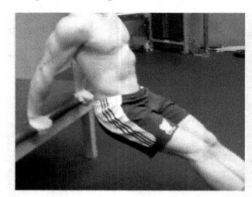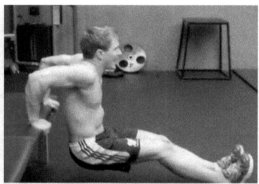

Fig 14. Triceps Bench Dips

Tip: If this exercise is too difficult, bring your feet back so they are closer to the chair or bench, for example, so your feet are just two feet in front. Or, only lower yourself partially during the descent.

Link to demonstration video: "How to: triceps bench dips. YouTube.

https://www.youtube.com/watch?v=c3ZGl4pAwZ4

Remember Rest and Recovery

At the risk of being repetitive, this is a reminder to give rest and recovery time their correct amount of attention if you want to optimize the results of your weightlifting and strengthening efforts. It can be tempting, especially when you are just getting started, to be enthusiastic and want to give it your all. It can be hard not to workout!

But, as you know by now, hypertrophy, the biological process that you will depend on to build muscles, is based on proteins and their component amino acids repairing and rebuilding the muscle cells and fibers damaged during lifting weights. Hypertrophy can only be functional when the muscles are allowed to rest for one or two days. At age 40-plus, two days is the preferable recovery time, and three days is even better.

Can You Lift Weights Every Day?

The answer to that question is both no and yes; it's a function of which muscles are being exercised on consecutive days:

➢ **No**, you should not exercise the same muscles or muscle groups on consecutive days. If you do chin-ups and barbell curls on Monday, your biceps and shoulders will not appreciate another round on Tuesday. The damage done to the muscles will not repair or grow to achieve over-rebuilding. Over time, what is medically called repeated insults will shrink the muscles and leave them weaker rather than stronger.

➢ **Yes**, if you work different muscles and muscle groups and allow the necessary rest time between workouts of the same muscles. For example, you could do the biceps and shoulders work on Monday, leg raises and squats on Tuesday, and then planks and seated cable rows on Wednesday, giving the biceps two full days to recover.

Can You Work Your Total Body?

While many weightlifters prefer shorter sessions, concentrating on a selective group of muscles, and getting their workouts done on five, six, or seven days each week, others prefer the alternative of working everything hard during one session, performing a complete routine of full-body exercises in a single workout session. During 40 or 50 minutes, they cover the arms and shoulders, chest and upper body, core, including the abdominals, back, upper and lower legs. So, the question is, can you, in middle-age, do this safely and productively?

> ➢ **Yes**, if it is done correctly and the need for rest and recovery is respected. You need to take two days of rest (or three) before repeating the full-body routine.
> ➢ Be aware that a total-body weightlifting workout takes longer than if you are concentrating on just two or three muscle groups. It can also be more of an exertion and can leave less experienced weightlifters exhausted.
> ➢ An advantage of fewer weightlifting sessions per week is that it leaves more days open for cardiovascular workouts. If you have allocated 40 or 45 minutes per day to work out, you can dedicate most of that time to running, fast walking, swimming, cycling, or hitting the elliptical and stair-climbing machines.
> ➢ Be sure to do light stretching before working out and then more stretching after the workout. We'll cover stretching in the next chapter.

When to Consult Your Doctor

In the spirit of "do no harm," as a middle-aged person who is beginning an exercise routine (or returning after a long layoff), it is important to take care of yourself and avoid injury. So should you see a doctor before beginning your workouts, or if you are experiencing pain or discomfort during or after exercise? The answer is yes to both questions.

See Your Doctor (1)

At this age, you should be having an annual physical exam with all of your vital signs checked out. Your doctor may refer you to a specialist, such as a cardiologist, to check your heart health, or an orthopedist if there are any joint or bone issues of concern. It's far better to confront potential problems early. It is normal and common for persons of middle-age to have aches and pains with the normal wear and tear of a life lived actively.

Even if you feel great and have no history of heart disease, getting your heart condition evaluated makes sense. A blood test will give a reading on a range of bodily conditions, and in particular, your doctor will probably check your blood lipids, which include HDL (good), LDL (bad) cholesterol, and triglycerides, and may even run an EKG to see your heart's electrical patterns. The doctor will listen carefully to your heartbeat and how your breathing is doing. A nurse will check your weight and blood pressure.

If you head to the cardiologist for a more in-depth analysis, you may take an exercise stress test to measure your heart's aerobic capacity or a CT scan to see how effectively your heart is pumping blood and if there are any arterial deposits. Rest assured that elevated levels of LDL cholesterol and triglycerides are easily treated today with inexpensive medications, notably statins, so don't put off getting checked out once you are age 40-plus. Hypertension (high blood pressure) is also potentially serious, yet treatable with a wide range of medications.

Your lifestyle should be evaluated, especially if you are overweight or obese, and the doctor may make dietary recommendations. (Chapter 6 will give you a good understanding of how to adopt a healthy diet.)

See Your Doctor (2)

There are many reasons that your workouts may prompt you to see your doctor, possibly having to do with heart-related concerns, or a joint, muscle, or tendon injury. Follow the warning that is posted on most aerobic exercise machines: if you feel pain in the chest, or become lightheaded, dizzy, or nauseous, stop and seek medical attention. It may be nothing, perhaps indigestion, or it may be a warning that something in your cardiovascular system needs prompt attention.

When the pain and discomfort in a joint are continuous and disruptive to normal activity, it is time to see the orthopedist, many of whom have training in sports medicine and are experienced with exercise-induced injuries. In many cases, you may be advised to follow the R.I.C.E. discipline: rest, ice, compression, and elevation. Certain joint injuries may require a cortisone injection to reduce inflammation and promote healing.

In summary, a little pain and discomfort is a normal result of lifting weights and working out. Use good sense when it comes to the amount of weight you are lifting, and be sure to respect the rest and recovery disciplines. Be alert to when the pain becomes serious, and do not ignore its warnings. The earlier that physical problems are diagnosed and treated, the faster the recovery.

Now, it's on to Chapter 5 with some more ideas about how to get your workouts going and keep them going.

Chapter 5

Metabolism, Motivation, Commitment

The objective of this chapter is to help you to understand what will make the difference in your being able to achieve the goals you are imagining for yourself as an aspiring weightlifter and fitness enthusiast. You may have tried weightlifting and bodybuilding before but gave it up as other responsibilities began to compete for your time and attention. Your energy level began to diminish, and you found the weights becoming heavier rather than lighter. You may have been a runner at one time, but that drifted away, too.

Or, this could all be new to you. You never (or almost never) lifted weights or did serious bodyweight calisthenics. Cardiovascular conditioning? No time, no interest?

No matter, you're here now and ready to step up to the challenges and rewards of getting more lean muscle, getting stronger, and being in overall good, healthy condition. You may be excited about getting started on the weightlifting and bodyweight calisthenics in the previous chapter, and that's great. But first, take a little time to understand why things are different for you now at middle-age, and why that is.

Continuity in your workouts and attention to your diet are essential, and they are for a reason beyond the basics of working out hard, getting adequate rest, and seeing positive results. As you age, things are slowing down, and muscle mass is diminishing. Why?

Metabolism: The Unseen Factor

Do you wonder why a person like yourself, who is middle-aged, cannot build muscle tissue and achieve bulk like someone in his 20s? Why does someone in their 40s lose muscle mass at a faster rate than someone in their 20s? Why does fat tend to build up more quickly, and why do the pounds add up even though you are eating the same amount as when you were younger? Now that you're age 40, 50, or more, there is an unseen factor that you need to understand and manage. It's your metabolism, the sum total of your body's biological and chemical cellular processing. At your age, it's slower than it used to be, and your fitness and dietary programs need to be adjusted to reverse the decline of your current metabolic rate.

Losing Muscle Mass

Lifestyle factors contribute to the slowing of your metabolism. You may be aware that most middle-aged people tend to follow a less active, more sedentary lifestyle that contributes to muscle loss, and it makes your commitment to a serious physical fitness routine much more important. But also, apart from your behavior, it is natural for you to experience muscle loss and the aging of your metabolic system.

Age-related muscle loss is called sarcopenia, and it is a normal, natural part of growing older. According to Harvard Health Publishing (2016), after age 30, you can lose from 3 percent to 5 percent of your muscle mass each decade. Men lose more muscle than women; on average 30 percent of their muscle mass disappears throughout their lifetimes.

But this degree of muscle loss is not inevitable, and muscle mass can be increased, rather than decreased, with a commitment to a good weightlifting program of resistance exercises that continues throughout middle-age.

Lost muscle mass can be recovered, according to Dr. Thomas W. Storer, director of Brigham and Women's Hospital's physical function and exercise physiology laboratory. He says that it takes work, planning, and dedication, but "it is never too late to rebuild muscle and maintain it" (2016).

The muscle loss, sarcopenia, is traced to declines in testosterone, and studies have been conducted to determine if testosterone supplements can slow or reverse muscle mass loss. While some results were positive, there were adverse effects, and the FDA has not approved testosterone supplements for building muscle mass in men.

As a result, Dr. Storer concludes that the optimal approach to building lean muscle mass, regardless of your age, is a continuing program of progressive resistance training: gradually increasing your workout volume by raising the amount of weight being lifted, and maintaining the number of reps and sets as your strength and endurance improve.

Metabolic Consumption Rates

Your metabolic rate directly affects the number of calories you burn in a day. This rate of caloric consumption is expressed in several ways:

➢ Your **resting** metabolic rate is measured when you are asleep, immobile, and resting and is the lowest rate that can sustain basic reflexes that keep you alive, including energy consumption to maintain your heartbeat, breathing, and brain functions. You burn the least number of calories per hour when in the resting state

➤ The **thermic** effect of food is the caloric consumption required to support digestion of the food you eat and process in a given period, including chewing and swallowing, grinding and acidification in the stomach, and the assimilation of food in the small and large intestines as it is carried through the GI tract by the contractions of peristalsis.

➤ **Non-exercise thermogenesis** includes all calories you burn while standing, sitting, writing, reading, speaking, laughing, doing light housework, and everything else that involves any physical effort except for exercise and digestion.

➤ **Exercise consumption** is the number of calories you burn during and immediately after exercise. This includes all active exercise, from walking to gardening, lifting and carrying, showering, stair climbing, jogging and running fast, weightlifting, swimming, and cycling, among other exertions.

The number of calories that are burned by these four categories varies from person to person based on individual metabolic rates and other factors, such as the type, amount, and intensity of the exercises and movements performed. Your metabolic rate can be affected by your age and certain physical characteristics such as muscle mass, height, weight, genetics, and hormones.

We'll get into calories and weight loss in the next chapter, but it's important to understand that weight gain, weight maintenance, and weight loss are entirely determined by two factors: the number of calories that are consumed and assimilated, and the number of calories that are metabolized. Any excess calories that exceed your daily needs and are not burned are stored as fat.

Raising Your Metabolism

Let's consider your metabolic control options. Can you influence the rate that your metabolism burns calories, especially since your metabolic rate is gradually declining with age? Exercise and other physical activities can have immediate positive effects on your metabolism and can also have a secondary effect during rest and even sleep:

> You can influence **non-exercise** thermogenesis by being a less sedentary, more active person, throughout the day. Walk instead of ride, take the stairs instead of the elevator, do your own housework, and fit some yoga stretching into your day (or Tai chi or Pilates), Avoid sitting as you work by arranging your laptop or desktop computer keyboard at a height that lets you work in a standing position at least part of the time. Over an average day, becoming more active and less sedentary can consume an additional 200, 600, or more calories as well as keeping you more flexible and healthier overall.

> **Exercise thermogenesis** can be an even more productive way to burn extra calories. The amount and intensity of the exercises are directly related to the calories, so, for example, a 40-minute weightlifting session can burn 500 to 600 calories compared to 40 to 80 calories consumed during that same time while sitting and watching TV or holding a conversation. Similarly, two miles on the

treadmill, either jogging or fast walking, can burn 200 to 220 calories in 20 to 30 minutes compared to 20 or so calories consumed while sitting.

➤ **Muscle gain:** Studies show that age-related metabolic slowdown is connected to the loss of muscle mass so that using weightlifting to build muscle mass will result in a greater overall metabolism rate even during the sleeping and resting phase, when the metabolic rate is at its slowest. A 10 percent increase in resting metabolism can result in several hundred incremental calories burned overnight with no exertion on your part!

The **most effective discipline** is to combine both of these practices: to be more active and less sedentary since this can increase your metabolism throughout the day; and to exercise with weightlifting and aerobics at least three days a week. You can't affect your metabolism based on how your body digests and absorbs foods, but adding more physical activity to your daily routine can turn up the caloric burn rate when you are taking it easy, even while sleeping.

Appetite effects: Here's a heads up to alert you to an effect on your weight that might surprise you It can cause you to gain more weight rather than losing or maintaining your current weight, despite your adoption of a weightlifting and aerobics program:

➤ While increasing your exercise regimen and daily rate of activity will burn more calories, it will probably also increase your appetite. This can lead to taking in more calories than you burn.

➤ Be careful not to snack excessively, and when you do snack or increase serving sizes at meals, emphasize lean protein, which will keep you feeling full longer (protein is slower to digest), and is beneficial to the muscle-building process of hypertrophy.

Motivation and Commitment

An important part of your long-term muscle and strength-building program is mental. Of course, it will be the weights, the reps, the sets, and the rests in between that will give you the lean muscle mass you want, but your state of mind will determine if you actually get started and if you will go the distance for the months and years of exercise it will take. Rome wasn't built in a day, and your impressive physique won't happen immediately.

The Motivation

In the initial chapter and at other points in this book, the importance of motivation was established as an incentive to getting your weightlifting and fitness program underway. No one can make you get into a regular, well-planned weightlifting program; you have to have the resolve and enthusiasm to take charge of your body, your health, and your appearance:

➢ If you have read this far, chances are good that you get it, "you're in."

➢ You imagine yourself lifting the barbells and dumbbells, doing the push-ups and pullups, the planks, the squats, and the splits.

➢ You feel committed to cardiovascular conditioning to help melt the extra pounds while you invest in your health and longevity.

➢ You feel better looking in the mirror in anticipation of the bigger, defined muscles you are going to build.

The Commitment

But will you have the determination and discipline to go the distance, to continue regularly with your bodybuilding and strengthening practices? Motivation is important at the beginning, but you need to have the discipline to stick to the routine even on days when you just don't have the drive, when you say, "I'll do it tomorrow."

You need to transcend the forces that hold you back, to break free of the constraints, and be committed no matter how tired or uninspired you are at that moment. Only then can you keep on track to meet your fitness and strengthening goals.

Commitment to succeed as a weightlifter, who builds muscle, who loses fat and excess weight, starts in the mind, which is the most effective and persuasive tool that will help you achieve your bodybuilding objectives. A positive attitude and the determination to work through the toughest movements will carry you through the worst of it with grit. Those who fail to make it, who give up, who quit, may be tough physically but don't have the mental toughness. Remember that your body will follow your mind.

Successful weightlifters at every level of training have developed positive thoughts to get themselves to the gym, to pick up the first weight of the session, to get through it with a full effort, no matter how tired or busy they were. You can adopt these thoughts, make them yours, let them carry you to the workout, and through the work, every time.

Positive Reinforcements

1. *I'll just do a half-workout today, take it easy.*

This works when you're tired and helps to get you started. In almost every case, once you get started and warmed up, you get into the movements, do all the reps, and go all the way. It's a little psychological game that you can play on yourself, and somehow it continues to work time after time. As it has been said, "just showing up is 90 percent of success," so just get those workout shoes and shorts on, get to a machine or a weight, and start out slowly. You'll warm up and keep going.

2. *The solo mountain climber's focus and discipline.*

When you are heading up the side of Yosemite's El Capitan, climbing without ropes or tools, there is no looking up or down, no thinking about what's coming or how hard it will be. The same applies to weightlifting when the only thing that matters is what you need to do at that moment: focus on the now. Another advantage of being in the moment while working out is the clearing of your mind, in a meditative way, so that all distractions are ignored. You will be calmer, and by paying close attention, your form and posture will be better, and you will be less likely to cause an injury.

3. *The mirror, the scale, and the tape measure.*

The numbers don't lie, exaggerate, or try to please your ego. They are the reality that will testify to the depth and duration of your commitment to building your body, getting your weight where it belongs, and getting that gut flatter. Start with a benchmark set of measurements, and check in every week. Look at yourself in the mirror without criticism or disappointment and just take notice of how your pecs (chest muscles) and abdominals look: a little soft, a layer of fat. Same for the arms and legs. Weigh yourself before breakfast, and write down the number each week, or daily if you prefer. Same for the tape measurement. Over time, you will see and record progress, and that will help solidify your commitment to your long-term objectives.

Inspirational Quotes

1. *"Tough times don't last, but tough people do."* — Richard Shuller (2020).

   This quote applies to all aspects of life but has found special appreciation among professional lifters who push to their absolute limits. But especially for you as you are beginning weightlifting and conditioning, there are times when it isn't fun, like that last pull-up or barbell curl. Your thighs may be burning after three sets of squats or splits, and that last set of dumbbell rows may have you breathing pretty hard. But every time the set is over, and the rest begins, the pain and burning feeling subsides, and the workout always ends with a feeling of work well done, a sense of satisfaction. You are tough and getting tougher.

2. *"To be a champion, you must act like a champion."* — Lou Ferrigno (2020).

   Lou Ferrigno, a champion weightlifter who played the Incredible Hulk, contributed to this recommended mindset because he believes that strength comes from within. A championship attitude is attainable by all of us if we believe in ourselves and envision the well-muscled, well-defined body we are working to achieve. But it goes further: If you want to become a well-built bodybuilder, you need to work out like one. Positive thinking is essential to motivate and inspire you, but without hard work and the determination to give it your all, positive thinking is just a dream.

3. *"Don't wish it were easier. Wish you were better."* — Jim Rohn (2020).

The thought leads us to expect that the workout, the lifting and pulling, the squatting and dipping, needs to be intensive, to challenge us. That leads to the realization that if it's easy, it's not being done right. You need to work to challenge your muscles to the point that muscle cells and fibers are damaged and need to self-repair through hypertrophy. The attitude that will carry you from passive to proactive is the recognition that it's a simple formula: strength is directly proportional to the effort that is invested in each workout. Of course, a hard workout can be followed in two days by a less intensive workout to aid recovery, but then be sure to make the next workout more intensive. It will pay off in the long-term.

4. *"It never gets easier. You just get stronger."* — Unknown (2020).

The idea is to add weights progressively when you can handle more without reducing reps, sets, or rest intervals. For example, head over to the dumbbell rack, and pick up a heavy weight you can do just one rep of a bicep curl or at most two. Do you wish you could do more reps? Find the weight you can lift or curl for eight reps and have the patience and confidence to know that in a reasonable time, with discipline, you will advance gradually from the lighter weight to the heavier ones and beyond. Just follow the basic practice of lifting weights that max out at eight to 10 reps, do the three sets, and be sure to rest between sets and between workouts.

5. *"You have to be at your strongest when you're feeling at your weakest."* — Unknown (2020).

This inspiration encourages weightlifters and cardio athletes to reach deep inside for the strength that they know is there. Imagine that you are a runner who is training for a marathon or other long-distance competition. The only time you can train is early in the morning before work, even in the cold and dark of winter. You need to roll out of bed at 5:30 a.m., wash your face, put on your running shoes, head outside, hit the road, and run into a biting cold headwind. What does it feel like to go through this, day after day, for months? This is what inner strength is all about, and it illustrates, in the extreme, what someone chooses to do to reach an objective. You probably will not have to work out under such an extreme condition. You'll be indoors, warm, lifting weights you can manage, and working to a reasonable, yet difficult peak of effort. But think of that runner in the dark, cold, early morning, and let it carry you to a better effort each day.

6. *"Strength does not come from physical capacity. It comes from an indomitable will."* — Mahatma Gandhi (2020).

The courage and determination that the leader of India's independence showed in standing up peacefully to overwhelming forces testify to the importance of resolve and commitment. Your willpower is what can help you accomplish what others think you cannot achieve. To friends, associates, and family, you may be wasting your time, risking injury, and for what? "You can't build muscles at your age," and "It's too late for you," they may say. Are they right? The answer is up to you. You can build muscle, get leaner and stronger, improve your health, well-being, and longevity if you have the will, the resolve to commit to a continuing program of progressive weightlifting, and aerobic training.

7. *"There are two types of pains, one that hurts you and the other that changes you."* — Unknown (2020).

A weightlifter's perspective. Too much pain can be harmful, but when you need to perform one more rep and the barbell feels like it weighs a ton, the discomfort of the extra effort that you need now won't last, but your satisfaction will. Too much pain can be dangerous, leading to injury and dampening your motivation to keep up with the regimen. But there is always some discomfort when you are trying to reach your peak output, and that is what you can expect, and need, to endure. The pain or strain you feel on the eighth or ninth rep won't hurt you; you are lifting or pulling the correct weight for your ability at that moment. It's the pain you feel on a first or second rep that is telling you the weight is too heavy for you, indicating you risk injury if you continue. Work progressively, and you will progress.

8. *"Pain is temporary. Quitting lasts forever."* — Lance Armstrong (2020).

The American prolific winner of the Tour de France has endured cycling up the mountains of the Alps and Massif Central while competing against the best bicyclists in the world. It was his resolve, his commitment, that kept him in the leader's yellow jersey to win seven successive tours. While nothing you will have to endure will approach the ordeal of a professional racer or weightlifter, you can learn and be inspired by their example. The intensity of their training is almost unimaginable, and frankly, the damage they are doing to their bodies can have long-term consequences. Don't try to imitate them, but let their "no quitting" attitude remind you on tough days that you will forget the momentary pain, discomfort, or inconvenience, but you may be disappointed in yourself if you don't go the distance.

Can you come up with your own quotes for motivation and commitment to building muscles and strength? All said, it's you who needs to be inspired, and no one knows you as well as you do. What makes you excited, enthusiastic, energized?

Now, a change of subjects. In Chapter 6, let's head into the kitchen and get the facts on how to eat better, healthier, and more satisfyingly to achieve your bodybuilding and strength building goals.

Chapter 6

Eating Right (and Loving It)

Eating Right in Middle-Age

The quality and composition of your diet are the most underrated aspects of physical fitness. Many people feel they have done the best they can for their fitness and health by spending hours every week in the fitness center or home gym, and they believe that gives them license to head into the kitchen and eat all they want of whatever they want. This is not correct.

There is truth to the adage, "you are what you eat," since your body is only able to assimilate and metabolize what you feed it. As you will see, a good diet will reward you in many ways, from keeping you leaner and helping to build muscles to giving you the energy and endurance you need to get stronger and get more done. Can your diet help you live longer? Yes, because a healthy diet will slow or stop the onset of heart disease, obesity, diabetes, chronic autoimmune disorders, gastrointestinal diseases, and degenerative diseases like Alzheimer's.

Your Three Essential Macronutrients

Nutritionists classify macronutrients as the three major food groups we've discussed: carbohydrates, proteins, and fats. These are separate from the many micronutrients like vitamins and minerals. There have been descriptions of the macronutrients in previous pages, but for clarity, let's get the definitions stated here. They are called "macro" because they are the larger amounts of food we eat, the totality of the calories we ingest, digest, assimilate, and metabolize.

Lindsey Wohlford, a wellness dietician at the MD Anderson Cancer Center, sums it up as the cornerstones of your diet:

> ➢ "Macronutrients are the nutritive components of food that the body needs for energy and to maintain the body's structure and systems" (2020).

Energy, structure, systems: the roles the macronutrients play are clearly defined.

Carbohydrates are your body's primary fuel, giving your muscles and your central nervous system the energy for movement, especially when the muscles are being worked or performing the exercise. According to Lindsey Wohlford, at least 45 percent and up to 65 percent of your daily caloric input should be from carbohydrates, or "carbs." We get our carbs from grains and cereals, fruits and vegetables, and foods containing sugar and other sweeteners. There is a popular misconception that carbohydrates are not good for us, but in reality, if they are from healthy sources like whole grains, fruits, and vegetables, and nuts and seeds, those are the essential carbs your body needs to keep going. There are four calories in one gram of carbs.

Protein is needed to give your body its structure, from muscles, ligaments, tendons, and bones, to skin and hair, organs, and nerves, down to cell membranes, and blood plasma. All are made from protein. Proteins are part of hormonal, enzyme, and metabolic systems and regulate the balance between acids and bases in your body. The recommended daily allowance (RDA) is 0.8 grams per kilogram of bodyweight, or 0.36 grams per pound, so a person weighing 150 pounds should consume about 50 grams of protein per day. However, when you are weightlifting to build muscles, your daily protein intake should be 75 grams or more. There are four calories in one gram of protein.

➤ The sources of protein in your diet are covered in detail later in this chapter.

Fats and oils (oils are fats that are liquid at room temperature) are your body's concentrated energy reserve and are higher in calories than the other two macronutrients. There are nine calories in one gram of fats, making storage easier. Stored fats can be called upon for energy when carbs (stored in the muscles as glycogen) are running low or depleted. Apart from energy, fats play a continuing role in providing insulation, protecting and cushioning your organs, and in the absorption and transport of fat-soluble nutrients, like vitamins D and E. The RDA for your daily fat consumption is between 20 percent and 35 percent of all calories, and saturated fats should be no more than 10 percent. Fats from extra virgin olive oil, avocados, and vegetable oils from soybeans, sunflower, safflower, and corn are monounsaturated or polyunsaturated and are recommended to promote cardiovascular health.

The 70:30 Rule of Fitness and Weight Management

Is achieving a high level of physical fitness and keeping your weight down attributable to 70 percent diet and only 30 percent physical training? The idea that diet is more than twice as important as working out has been popular among trainers and athletes for some time, but there does not appear to be a scientific basis for this precise ratio, although it is heading in the right direction. There is scientific evidence to show there are limits to how much exercise alone can contribute to weight loss.

As reported in the Guardian (2016), while exercise is definitely important for your health and well-being, research indicates that physical activity alone will not necessarily consume extra calories:

> ➢ Leading to the conclusion that diet should be the primary tactic to achieve weight loss.

This is based on studies that show that our metabolic processes reach a plateau beyond which additional exercise, whether it's weightlifting, cardio or both, does not continue the same rate of energy expenditures. Beyond a certain point, the body makes adjustments to constrain, or limit, how many calories are burned in a given time.

For example, after a day that included a long, intensive weightlifting and cardio workout from which you burned 650 extra calories, your metabolism may slow down more than normal while you're resting and asleep so your net calorie loss for the day is only 150 to 250 calories. Other studies reported in Current Biology (2016), which involved humans and other primates, showed that those who performed extra physical activity did not burn substantially more calories in 24 hours than those who performed moderate activity, but both groups did burn more calories than sedentary individuals whose activity levels were low.

At City University of New York, Professor Herman Ponzer, who participated in the study, said, "Exercise is really important for your health," but went further to conclude:

> ➢ "What our work adds is that we also need to focus on diet, particularly when it comes to managing our weight and preventing or reversing unhealthy weight gain" (2016).

Diet plays a larger role in maintaining a healthy weight and providing the essential nutrients for building muscle, maintaining a healthy metabolism, managing weight, and keeping a strong immune system to keep out disease and the incursions of aging.

Your body's health and strength, as well as your energy and endurance, are dependent upon the fuel you ingest and the quality and types of foods you eat. As important as weightlifting is to building muscles, and you're becoming stronger and more fit, your diet is as influential, possibly more so. In recognizing that our diet plays a key role in building muscle and keeping off fat, we'll help you cut through all the dietary misinformation and get you pointed to a lifelong dietary practice rather than a series of fad diets that come and go. There are fundamentals of nutrition that you will learn to follow.

Calories In, Calories Out

It's called the CICO diet, but it's not really a diet; it's a basic law of science. It stands for Calories In, Calories Out, and it means that weight maintenance is based on digesting the same number of calories that you burn each day. There are 3,500 calories in one pound of bodyweight, so if you wanted to lose one pound per week, you would have to take in 500 fewer calories than you burn each day in each week. The amount you burn is based on your unique metabolic rate, your activity level, and what you have ingested since certain foods are digested more readily and more completely than others.

➢ As you have just read in the previous section, exercise alone will not burn as many calories as you'd think.

➢ The way to improve the ratio of CICO is to take in fewer calories.

A calorie is simply a unit of energy. There are four calories in one gram of carbohydrate, four calories in a gram of protein, but nine calories in a gram of fat, which is nature's efficient way of storing energy and why foods that are high in fats and oils are, well, fattening.

Satiety: Feeling Full

One of the ways certain foods can be less or more fattening is their satiety level. The amount of fullness you feel slows how hungry you become and want to eat again. In general, foods that are high in protein are better at keeping you full longer because the complex protein molecules are harder for your digestive system to break down into their amino acid building blocks and then assimilate. This compares to the less complex molecules that compose carbohydrates and fats, which pass through the stomach and are digested much more quickly.

But even certain foods in the same categories have different satiety levels. A serving of boiled potatoes has the same number of calories from carbohydrates as a French pastry, like a croissant, but the potatoes are seven times more filling, research shows. This may be due to the carbohydrates in potatoes being composed of complex starches, which are slow to break down, and the croissant being made from two highly refined carbohydrates: white flour and sugar. It also contains butter, which also digests quickly.

The refined ingredients in the croissant illustrate the concerns that nutritionists have with highly refined and processed foods. Writing in Today (2020), registered dietician Samantha Cassetty says that instead of focusing just on calories:

➢ "It's better to be aware of your calorie needs and to develop an understanding of how calories from various foods make you feel."

➢ Controlling your appetite "with filling foods that are also in line with your body's calorie needs is a good way to manage your weight and your hunger levels," she concludes.

Limiting Highly Processed Foods

Highly processed foods account for about 60 percent of the average American diet and are blamed for adding excess calories, sodium (salt), chemical additives (for preservation, flavor enhancement, and color), saturated fats, and refined sugar. In consequence, this type of diet leads to weight gain, elevated levels of LDL (bad) cholesterol, high blood pressure, and higher blood sugar levels.

A small scale study reported in Cell Metabolism (2019) dramatically demonstrates the differences between a diet of highly processed foods and one of whole, unprocessed foods. Twenty participants first spent two weeks eating a processed diet exclusively, followed by the natural, unprocessed, whole foods. Both diets were matched with equal quantities of carbohydrates, protein, fats and oils, and fiber. Importantly, during the study, the participants were allowed to eat as much or as little as they wanted.

At the end of the study, the findings included:

> ➢ On the processed diet, participants ate an average of 500 calories per day more than on the whole foods diet and gained two pounds.

> ➢ When the same people switched to the unprocessed whole foods diet, they lost two pounds.

> ➢ It was noted that during the processed diet phase, participants ate faster and ate more, suggesting that the processed foods were less filling and signals of satiation were slower to reach the brain.

> ➢ It is also possible that faster and excessive eating was encouraged by higher amounts of salt and flavor enhancements in processed foods.

Conclusions include the reality that extra calories, regardless of the source, lead to weight gain, and further, it is postulated that unrefined, unprocessed foods, especially grains, are slower to be digested and absorbed, possibly due to high fiber content, and also raise resting metabolism rates.

The Importance of Protein in Middle-Age

Our bodies need carbohydrates, protein, and fats, but as a middle-age weightlifter aspiring to build muscle mass, your need for protein is greater than normal because you need that protein to build muscle tissue and to enable hypertrophy to function effectively. Being older, that need for protein is even greater.

Protein has specific benefits that benefit all people, but especially when you are middle-aged and want to pursue a physically active lifestyle.

1.   **Weight loss** through appetite and hunger control. As noted, protein is slower to digest than carbohydrates and fats. It takes longer for the stomach acids and enzymes to break it down, so it stays there longer. There are weight-regulating hormonal factors as well:

➢ Ghrelin is a hunger stimulant that is suppressed by protein. This may be the result of the protein digesting slowly, causing the stomach to send a signal to the brain to slow down the release of ghrelin as if to say, "full house, no room here."

➢ Protein also invites the release of YY peptide, which is a hunger suppressant. It makes you feel full and less likely to reach for something else to eat.

In a study among overweight women, the participants increased their protein intake from 15 percent to 30 percent, and on average they consumed 441 fewer calories per day. That could cause the loss of one pound every eight days. The quantity of protein needed to reach 30 percent of a 2,000-calorie-per-day diet is equal to 600 calories, or 150 grams.

2.   **Reduced late-night snacking** is another result of the" feeling fuller longer" effect of slow digesting protein and the ghrelin and YY peptide appetite suppression effects. A study among overweight men, in which protein intake was increased to 25 percent of total calories, showed late-night cravings were reduced by 60 percent and the desire to snack at night was lowered by 50 percent.

3.   **The building block of muscle.** Muscle cells and fibers are constructed of protein, during hypertrophy, when the muscle cells and fibers are being repaired following the damage that occurs during a weightlifting workout, protein is the "brick

and mortar" that is piled on and patched in. Insufficient protein in the diet will retard hypertrophy and can lead to muscle loss.

> As an aspiring middle-age weightlifter, you need to be aware that your need for protein is greater than for those who are a decade or two youngers. Your repair mechanisms and metabolism are slower and need more "raw materials" to patch up the damaged protein within your muscles.

4.   **Bones need protein, too.** With age comes bone porosity, leading to osteoporosis and the risk of broken bones. While we think of calcium as the key component of bones (it is), protein plays an important role in helping to reinforce the calcium so that the bones are harder and less porous. This refutes the misconception that protein makes bones more fragile by leaching away the calcium; it's simply not true.

5.   **Faster metabolism and fat-burning.** Eating and the process of digestion burns calories and fat because work is being done and energy is being expended. This process is called the thermic effect of food, and it varies depending on the food being digested. Protein's thermic effect is four times greater than when carbohydrates or fats are being digested, so it boosts metabolism and burns more calories. In one study, the higher protein diet burned about 100 more calories, and in another study that compared a high-protein group with a low-protein group, the net caloric burn for the high protein group was 260 calories per day.

6.   **Helps protect against heart disease.** Analysis of 40 different studies of increased protein in the diet found that systolic blood pressure (top number) was lowered by 1.76 mm Hg, and diastolic pressure (bottom, smaller number) was lowered by 1.15 mm Hg. There was also a lowering of LDL (bad) cholesterol and triglycerides. These findings suggest a higher

protein diet can help prevent strokes, heart attacks, and chronic kidney diseases.

7.   **Speeds recovery after injury.** When you are injured, most of the damage is done to your skeletal muscles, which are made of protein, and those muscles need protein to repair themselves. Bone damage needs protein to speed repairs. A higher protein diet also increases platelets in the blood, which are used to clot and stop bleeding.

8.   **Maintaining your fitness as you age.** A natural consequence of aging is the weakening of your muscles and reduction in muscle mass. The combination of increased protein in the diet and resistance exercises has been confirmed to prevent the onset of sarcopenia, which is age induced muscle loss and deterioration. The exercise will encourage rebuilding and muscle growth, but adequate amounts of protein need to be available to allow hypertrophy to operate effectively.

Sources of Protein

The following are excellent sources of protein with additional muscle-building and health benefits. We begin with dairy and egg protein sources, then fish and seafood, then meat and plant sources.

Dairy and Egg Protein Sources

Greek yogurt is higher in protein than regular yogurt because it is strained to remove some of the water, thus concentrating what is left. There are 16 to 19 grams of protein in a ¾-cup serving, which is double that of regular yogurt. The protein in Greek yogurt is a combination of fast-digesting whey protein and slow-digesting casein protein. There is further benefit from the live probiotic bacteria cultures, which support the microbiome in the gut. Greek-style, high-protein yogurt is also available as Icelandic or Australian yogurt. Check the labels to be sure about the protein content. Choose low-fat or fat-free versions to save on calories and avoid saturated fats.

Milk is a good source of protein and carbohydrates, and while it can contain up to 4 percent partially saturated fats, there are low-fat and fat-free versions that are abundantly available (and recommended vs. full fat). The protein in milk, as in yogurt, contains both fast- and slow digesting proteins, which are thought to contribute to muscle building and muscle cell and fiber enhancement. Studies show that consumption of milk after hard workouts resulted in more muscle growth compared to the same workouts followed by carbohydrates.

Cottage cheese is a concentrated source of protein with 28 grams in a one-cup, eight-ounce serving. Like other dairy sources, cottage cheese protein is high in the muscle-building amino acid, leucine. And as with milk and dairy, you may choose from fat-free, low-fat, or full-fat versions. As dairy fats tend to be high in saturated fats, you are encouraged to opt for the fat free or low-fat versions.

Eggs provide quality protein with one egg containing six grams of protein, and only 70 calories. Eggs are high in the amino acid leucine, which is a key muscle-building component of protein. Eggs have additional nutritional benefits, including choline and B vitamins, and are recommended to be eaten despite containing cholesterol. If you prefer, increase your consumption of egg whites, which are cholesterol-free and almost pure protein.

Fish and Seafood Protein Sources

Salmon is a cold-water fish that is high in omega-3 fatty acids, which provide antioxidant benefits and are believed to contribute to muscle growth. There are 34 grams of protein in a six-ounce serving of lean salmon steak. Canned salmon is similarly high in protein and nutrients. Other Coldwater fish like cod, sea bass, turbot, mackerel, and sardines are also recommended as is tuna, discussed next.

Tuna is even a bit higher in protein than salmon, with 40 grams in a six-ounce serving, plus vitamin A and B vitamins, including B6, B12, and niacin, all of which contribute to energy and workout performance. Tuna also has a high level of antioxidant omega-3 acids, which are believed to slow the rate of age-related muscle loss. As with salmon, canned tuna is similarly high in protein and nutrients, compared with fresh.

Shrimp is another high-protein seafood choice, with 36 grams of protein in a six-ounce serving. Shrimp are high in the muscle-building amino acid leucine. With minimal fats and virtually no carbohydrates, a six-ounce serving of shrimp contains only 144 calories.

Scallops are almost identical to shrimp in their nutritional composition but are a little higher in calories and protein with 40 grams in a six-ounce serving.

Meat Protein Sources

Chicken breast, served lean with skin removed and any visible fat cut away, is very high in protein with 26 grams of pure protein in a three-ounce serving or 52 grams in a six-ounce piece. There are also good amounts of vitamins B6 and niacin, which are credited with helping your body functioning during exercise and creating favorable conditions for muscle growth.

Lean beef is close to chicken breast in providing a high level of protein, but the challenge is to select beef that is truly low in fat. Avoid fatty cut by choosing a lean steak and cut away all visible fat. Avoid cuts that are marbled with fat that cannot be removed. When using ground beef, select the 95 percent lean option, which is far lower in saturated fat calories: a three ounce serving of 95 percent lean beef contains 145 calories compared to 228 calories for 70 percent lean beef.

Turkey breast is very lean white meat, and when served without skin (which may contain a layer of fat), it provides 25 grams of protein in a three-ounce serving. The 100 calories in this serving are almost all fat and carbohydrate-free, and like chicken breast, high in musclebuilding B vitamins, especially niacin.

Plant Sources of Protein

There are a few plant-based foods that contain a complete protein with the nine essential amino acids we need in our diets, but most plant sources are incomplete and need to be supplemented by other plant-based sources that are complementary:

> ➤ A combination of beans, legumes, and grains provide all necessary amino acids for nutritionally complete protein.
> ➤ For example, a meal made with black, pinto, or kidney beans, combined with brown rice or wheat-based pasta, provides nutritionally complete protein.

> However, protein levels in animal-derived foods are far more concentrated and provide more protein per ounce or measure compared to plant-sourced protein.

Soybeans are probably the best-known plant source of complete protein with good reason. There are 14 grams of protein in ½-cup of cooked soybeans with beneficial unsaturated fats, vitamin K, and the important minerals, iron and phosphorus. You may also choose immature fresh or frozen soybeans, called edamame. One cup of edamame beans contains 17 grams of protein and eight grams of fiber, which aids digestion. It contains significant amounts of manganese and vitamin K, plus folate, which is credited with helping to process amino acids and optimize muscle growth among middle-aged and older people.

Quinoa is a grain that has complete, or nearly complete, protein, plus a large amount of unrefined, healthy carbohydrates for energy. One cup of cooked quinoa contains eight grams of protein, along with 40 grams of carbohydrates and five grams of digestion-supporting fiber. Its nutrients include phosphorus and magnesium, which aids the function of the nervous system's coordination with skeletal muscles.

Beans, including kidney, lima, black, and pinto, are a good source of vegetative-source protein with 15 grams of protein in one cup of cooked beans. As noted above, beans need to be paired with grains and cereals, like rice, oats, quinoa, wheat, and rye (in bread or pasta, for example). Beans are rich in nutrients, including B vitamins and the minerals iron, phosphorus, and magnesium.

Other nutritional plant sources of protein include brown rice, oats, chickpeas, peanuts, almonds, and buckwheat (used in baking instead of flour). Grains and cereals are lower than beans and legumes in protein and higher in carbohydrates. Nuts are higher than most foods in oils, which are unsaturated and beneficial, but high in calories, so be careful how many you eat.

Is There an Ideal Diet?

Walk into a bookstore and look for the section for books on diet. You will need time just to read the titles because the number of diets that are recommended is extensive. There are several reasons for this:

> ➤ Many people need help and guidance on weight loss and for managing conditions and illnesses: diabetes, heart disease, hypertension, cancers, immune disorders, and psychological problems among others.
> ➤ There is generally a belief that there is a magic diet, a silver bullet solution to lose weight, build muscle, cure disease, and live longer.
> ➤ Diet is all about eating, and people generally take eating very seriously as evidenced by the size of the cookbook section at the bookstore.

Let's take a quick look at some of the diets that are popular today, but with the understanding that while there are responsible ways to help with weight control and prevent or alleviate certain diseases, there is no single amazing diet that is the solution for everyone's problems. There is no "one size fits all" die because each of us has our own unique physiology, our own metabolic rate, our own sensitivities.

Popular Diets

Fasting has emerged recently as a way to health, happiness and a longer life, but you need to know that while the research involving worms and mice has been encouraging, the studies involving humans are mostly in the early stages. The more common approaches are intermittent fasting, conducted on a daily, repeating basis, such as the 16:8 fasting diet, which allows eating during an eight-hour period (e.g., 8 a.m. to 4 p.m.), and nothing to eat for the next 16 hours (4 p.m. to 8 a.m.). There are stricter versions, like 18:6. Alternatively, some try prolonged fasting, going for 24- or even 48- hour fasts, followed by a day of unlimited eating. People who practice this tend not to overeat on the non-fast days because their stomachs shrink a bit during the fast period,

➤ As a weightlifter seeking to build muscles, fasting diets are not advised for you.

Paleo diets harken back to paleolithic, simpler times when our distant ancestors were hunter gatherers and ate "off the land," which means whatever they could find. This inspires diets today that avoid all refined and processed foods (which is commendable) and based on foods that our bodies evolved over millions of years to digest effectively.

According to the Mayo Clinic, a paleo diet usually includes vegetables, fruits, nuts and seeds, lean meats, and fish, which are the foods that could be gained by hunting and gathering. A paleo diet limits foods like dairy products, grains and legumes, and potatoes that became available when farming and agriculture started around 10,000 years ago. Added salt is also avoided. Overall, the paleo diet is acknowledged as healthy and wholesome as long as the ratios of macronutrients are respected, and a diversity of foods is included so that adequate amounts of vitamins and minerals are included.

Keto diet, short for ketogenic, has a very specific objective: rapid weight loss through stimulation of fat burning. This is achieved by following a very high-fat, very low-carbohydrate diet, essentially replacing the carbs with fats. This results in a metabolic condition called ketosis, which is highly efficient in using stored and dietary fat, instead of carbs and stored glycogen, for energy. You burn fat; you lose weight. Another quality is the conversion of fat stored in the liver to ketones, which supply energy to the brain. Also, the keto diet has been shown to lower blood sugar and insulin levels, which may contribute to the prevention or reduction of diabetes and other disorders. Other benefits are a feeling of fullness (satiety) that reduces cravings to eat or snack and improved mood. Studies of the longer-term effects of keto and other very low-carb diets are underway.

While the keto diet appears to be effective for weight loss, it may not include sufficient protein for building muscle mass; at least 30 percent of your diet should be protein.

Mediterranean diet. Let's conclude with a diet that is not only gaining broad acceptance, but it is the closest to the ideal diet everyone is searching for. It includes a wide range of wholesome and great-tasting foods, is affordable, is credited by the medical community as being heart-healthy, and may help slow the onset of many other diseases, from diabetes to cancer.

This diet is based on the practices of long-term residents of the Mediterranean Basin, including parts of Italy, Spain, and France, who tend to live healthier, longer lives. But importantly, these people practice a lifestyle that includes not only diet, but also being physically active all their lives, keeping their weight at normal levels, and having a positive attitude towards life.

The components of the Mediterranean diet:

➤ A variety of fresh vegetables, fresh and dried fruits, nuts, and seeds, whole grains and cereals, fish, lean meat in small servings (e.g., six ounces), moderate quantities of dairy (mostly as cheese), eggs, extra virgin olive oil, and wine, mostly red, consumed in moderation.

Whatever diet you choose, remember that as a weightlifter and builder of strength and muscle, you need sufficient protein in your diet, and you should select foods that are low in saturated fats. Avoid salty, processed foods, fried foods, and anything containing large amounts of sugar. The next section details the good and bad sources of foods.

Food Sources: Good and Bad

The types and sources of the three macronutrients have been discussed in detail, but to summarize, here is a quick checklist of the good and the bad. While this chapter has been devoted to helping you to understand the foods that are most beneficial to your health and to improve your level of physical fitness, build muscle and make you stronger, there are sources of carbohydrates, proteins, and fat that you should avoid. To help your dietary planning, we've listed both the recommended sources of your macronutrients and the foods that have been designated as undesirable and potentially harmful.

According to nutritionists at MD Anderson Cancer Center:

Recommended carbohydrates sources include:

➤ Dairy products, including milk, yogurt, and cottage cheese, but with a preference for low-fat or non-fat since full-fat dairy products are high in saturated fats and calories. Non-dairy substitutes made from soy, almonds, and oats are also good sources of carbs. Dairy products also provide high-quality complete protein.

➤ Vegetables, which can be eaten without limitation since they are low in calories and rich in vitamins and minerals. Select a variety of colors (green, yellow, red, purple) which will provide a diversity of micronutrients.

➤ Fruits are high in natural sugars (which is why they taste sweet) and micronutrients. Fruit should be eaten without added sugar and in natural, solid form to preserve pulp, which adds valuable fiber. Many juices have added sugar and the pulp has been removed.

➤ Beans, peas, and lentils, known as legumes, provide high levels of carbohydrates, plus fiber and many of the 20 amino acids that comprise protein.

➤ Whole grains, including whole wheat, rye, buckwheat, spelt, corn, and oats, are high in carbs and are excellent sources of vitamin B and fiber. Refined grains do not have these added qualities.

Carbohydrate sources to avoid:

➤ Refined flours and sugar, found in crackers, most breads, cookies, breakfast cereals, and sugar, in most fruit juices, soft drinks, most athletic performance beverages, and candy.

Recommended protein sources include:

➤ Beans, including black, pinto, and kidney beans, plus lentils and soy products. Except for soy, the proteins are incomplete and need supplementation with grains and cereals.

➤ Nuts and seeds, including nut butters (sugar-free versions).

➤ Whole grains, including quinoa, rye, wheat, spelt, corn, and soy, with the caveat that the amino acids do not comprise complete protein.

➤ Animal protein from meat, poultry, fish and seafood, dairy, and eggs.

Protein sources to avoid:

➤ Processed meats, like sausages, salami, bacon, frankfurters (hot dogs), and canned lunch meats.

➤ Consumption of lean red meats should be limited to 18 ounces per week.

Recommended fat sources include:

➤ Vegetable oils, especially extra virgin olive oil, avocado oil, and canola oil, and secondarily, oils from corn, sunflower, and safflower.

➤ Fatty fish, notably cold-water salmon, tuna, mackerel, and sardines.

➤ Flax seeds, chia seeds, avocados, and olives.

➤ Nuts and seeds, and again, natural nut butters, no sugar added.

Fat sources to avoid:

> ➤ Fried foods, which are made with refined flour and absorb large amounts of oils that contain trans fats.
> ➤ Animal sources, including full-fat dairy like milk, butter, yogurt, cream cheese, and the fats on meats and poultry.
> ➤ Vegetable oils from coconut and palm sources, shortening (used in baking), soft tub margarines, and most packaged baked goods (read the labels for fat content).

Now, on to Chapter 7 and dismissing some common misconceptions about working out, getting into shape, building muscles, and gaining strength when you are 40-plus.

Chapter 7

Common Misconceptions About Fitness After 40

What to believe? You are middle-aged and about to begin a serious strengthening and fitness program. Is it safe? Should you be doing this at your age? Maybe you've been warned by others or have concerns of your own. Let's get to the facts.

1. You're too old to be lifting weights and doing cardio workouts.

Let's put this myth to bed quickly. There is no age limit to becoming fit. If you are male or female, age 40, 50, or 60, you actually need a good exercise program more now than when you were younger. Yes, it would have been easier when you had the muscles and arteries of a 20year-old, but in those days, your body took care of itself. Now your metabolism is slower, the fat tends to accumulate more easily, and you are losing muscle mass. Your bones may be getting more porous and susceptible to breakage. A good resistance and aerobics program can reverse those symptoms of aging. If you're new to this and out of shape, see your doctor first, as we advise in Chapter 4, get the proper cautions, then get to work bringing your body back to its fitness and health potential.

2. You need to spend more time working out.

Being middle-age is not a rationale for extending your workouts. Less is more when you perform an intense, quality workout, so there's no basis for overdoing it or wasting time you may need elsewhere. Even when time precludes a full workout at the health club, you can still spend 20 minutes at home giving yourself a good workout with weights or by doing bodyweight calisthenics. Even when there's no time pressure, a complete weightlifting or cardiovascular workout can be done in 40 minutes or less. Any more than that may lead to overwork injuries, especially in middle age, so control your time to optimize the workout.

3. You should not do high-intensity workouts.

It all depends what is meant by intensity. For weightlifting, there is overwhelming evidence that you can build muscle in middle-age as long as you work up to your peak levels gradually and find the sweet spot between too little weight and too much. Here's a reminder of the recommendations in the book. After warming up, perform between eight and 10 reps with weights you can just make to those last one or two reps. If you can't do more than less than eight, it's too heavy, and if you can do more than 10, the weight is too light. Do three sets of eight to 10 reps with the optimal weight and your workout will have all the intensity you need.

4. You do not have time to workout.

Maybe you are at a point in your career when it's all on the line, and you need to get to work early and stay late. You feel that 30 or 40 minutes out of your day just isn't affordable to you. Recalling Parkinson's law that work expands to fill the available time, you should re-evaluate your work ethic; you may realize that you do have more discretionary time. Ask yourself if you really don't have the time or is it that you don't have the motivation to exercise, get stronger, and be fit? If you've jumped to this chapter before reading the book, head back to Chapter 5 and read about motivation and commitment. You also have the option to break up your workouts to a few minutes here and there throughout the day, getting up and moving around. Studies confirm that you can burn the calories, challenge the muscles, and strengthen the heart in short bursts.

5. Running is dangerous and should be avoided.

Running at middle-age does have some risks. especially for your joints, and connective tissues, so we need to find the ideal, safe way to run. Ideally, you can run on a treadmill, which cushions your steps, and is far less likely to bother your knees, which are the most susceptible to wear and tear as the years go by. If you do want to run outdoors, try for softer surfaces like grass or trails through forests and parks. Wear a good pair of running shoes to cushion and also prevent your foot from pronating, or rolling. If running becomes painful, consider switching to race walking, which doesn't pound the joints, yet can give you a good cardio workout.

6. Either diet or exercise will keep weight down, you don't need both.

This is covered in Chapter 6, but to hit the key points: diet is by far the more influential in managing your weight. Calories in, calories out (how many calories you digest vs. how many you burn) is the prevailing scientific principle, and it is far easier to resist ingesting the 500calorie pair of iced doughnuts or a cup of full-fat ice cream than to have to run or walk five miles to burn those calories off. Especially since studies prove that calories burned through exercise are partially offset by a slower metabolism when you're resting or asleep. The best way to lose weight is to follow a responsible diet (not a fad diet) and eat less while you continue your fitness program. Increase the protein in your diet to better build muscles, keep you fuller longer, and less likely to snack.

7. It's too late to lose belly fat.

The same "calories in, calories out" principle applies here as well. If you burn more calories in a given period than you consume and digest, your weight will go down, and excess fat will be what is lost. Now, it's true that fat tends to accumulate around your gut as you get older and your metabolism slows down. But even that fat can't stay for long if you maintain a good caloric deficit. Unfortunately, we can't "spot reduce" fat, meaning abdominal exercises like leg raises and planks, will harden the muscles but will have no direct effect on the belly fat. If you want to lose fat, the best approach is to lose weight through a combination of diet and exercise.

Conclusion

This book was written for anyone who is over age 40 and is thinking that it's time to get into good physical shape, either for the first time or to return to the good condition of when you were younger. If you are concerned that it may be too late for you, that you've waited too long to begin or to resume working out, this book assures you that it's not too late, In fact, your timing is excellent.

Let's recap by reviewing the key points of what the book has covered.

Your body has evolved. It is no longer the body of when you were 20 or even 30; your metabolism is slowing, imperceptibly but gradually, year after year, and you have been losing muscle mass, and gaining fat. These changes may be obvious, or subtle, but they are happening as a natural part of the aging process. But these changes are not inevitable and can be slowed, stopped, or even reversed by a well-planned fitness program involving weightlifting and other resistance exercises, cardiovascular conditioning, and a responsible diet.

Stronger after 40? Can you really build muscles and get stronger after 40? Yes, because there is science behind the workouts, the sweat, and exertion. It's called hypertrophy, the process of tearing down muscle cells and fiber while lifting weights, and then resting while your body repairs the damage by adding protein and overbuilds slightly. Over time, the overbuilding accumulates, creating larger, stronger muscles. This process may happen more slowly at age 40 or 50, but it happens nonetheless.

> ➤ You can exercise hard, just not the same old way.
> ➤ Your age is not a barrier to achieving serious muscle bulk and definition once you learn how to perform the right exercises with the right weights and routines.

Lifting heavy weights. The question of how much weight to lift safely, yet effectively, leads to options from many reps of light weights to very few — one, two, or three — reps that you can barely handle. The optimal weights are those you can lift eight to 10 times with the last rep being really tough to lift, pull, or push all the way. So, yes, you can lift heavy weights as long as you follow the eight-to-10 reps maximum.

Motivation, commitment, consistency. A successful muscle-building, strength, and fitness program requires the motivation to begin, but even more importantly, you need an unshakeable commitment to consistently renew your dedication to weightlifting and cardiovascular training over the long term:

> ➤ Without motivation, getting started might be put off indefinitely, or you may start your workouts half-heartedly. But motivation is only the stimulus, the catalyst to get you started; it's commitment and consistency that will drive you to achieve your muscle-building and fitness goals. Without commitment and consistency in your progressive training, you may be tempted to quit or slow down, and that will not get you where you need to go.
> ➤ Begin every day with a self-image of who you want to be. Picture those bigger biceps, the well-defined chest and abdominals, the powerful legs, the flat gut. Resolve every morning, as soon as you wake up, to achieve that body, that strength, vitality, and energy.

> ➤ Consistency requires willpower, and you know you have it deep within. You can call on it to pull on those gym shorts and workout shoes every day and give your muscles and your heart the conditioning they need and deserve as you renew your effort and commitment to longevity and health.

> ➤ Consider each workout to be an investment in long-term physical equity. Like building a solid wall, a few bricks and mortar at a time, hypertrophy slowly but consistently increases muscle tissue. Commit to long-term growth.

> ➤ Progress may be slow at middle-age, imperceptible on a daily or weekly basis, but by making your workouts a continuing routine over the months and years, your commitment to consistency will pay off with the body you dream of. Slow progress is better than no progress, and with tenacity and patience, great results will be there for you.

> ➤ Your workouts will vary in their intensity, and some days will feel fulfilling and other days less so. But there are no bad workouts — showing up is what it takes — because the only "bad" workout is the one you didn't do. Remember the tip: on days when it's tough to even think about working out, tell yourself you'll just take it easy with a few dumbbell lifts, a few push-ups, but know that once you get started and warmed up, your energy will return and you'll put in a good workout.

You can do this. This book has you covered with ways to get started and maintain your commitment and resolve to reach your muscle, strength, and fitness objectives. You have seen the workouts of celebrity athletes, from James Bond to The Rock, and while you are not going to follow their extreme workouts, you can be inspired by their examples of dedication and discipline.

Do no harm. In presenting a range of weightlifting exercises and calisthenics, you have noted the upfront warning of do no harm and be respectful of your age and your body. Warm up and start slowly with weights more on the lighter side until you get the hang of it.

Where to workout? You may have access to a well-equipped health club, fitness center, or gym and will be able to use free weights, exercise machines with cables to pull and handles to push, plus rubber stretch bands (which can replicate many weight and machine movements), and treadmill and elliptical machines for cardiovascular workouts. Or you may want a home gym with some free weights, like dumbbells and barbells, rubber stretch bands and tubes, and a bar for pull-ups and chin-ups.

Another good option, which requires almost no equipment, is bodyweight calisthenics, which you can perform at home or anywhere. Your bodyweight actually can provide quite a lot of resistance; think of how much weight you are lifting when you do push-ups, squats, or pullups.

Full-body workout. The seven weightlifting and seven calisthenics exercises are more than enough for you to achieve full-body workouts challenging every muscle group. You are encouraged to draw your routines from both groups if you have the weights; otherwise, you can achieve equally impressive results entirely with bodyweight calisthenics. Each exercise includes a link to a video demonstration with good instructions from professional trainers so you can learn and perform the movements safely and effectively.

Rest and recovery. You have been instructed in the importance of rest and recovery since the process of hypertrophy takes time, and even more as you get older. Muscle groups should have at least one day of rest, preferable two, between resistance workouts. You have the choice of working the full body and resting for two or three days, or working out more frequently and limiting each workout to one or two muscle groups, like arms and shoulders on Monday, chest and core on Tuesday, legs on Wednesday, and back to arms and shoulders on Thursday. You have the freedom to select the routines and timing that work for you. You should aim to work each muscle group at least two times each week.

Metabolic rate. You've received a briefing on your metabolism to understand what it is, how it affects your bodily functions, and why and how it slows as the years pass. The importance of being highly motivated to start your strengthening and fitness program is again emphasized as is the need for the commitment to keep your fitness program going over the long term, making it a valued component of your lifestyle. Hopefully, the inspirational quotes in that section will give you added drive.

You are what you eat. The subject of diet was covered in detail and sought to bring clarity to the often-misunderstood role of carbohydrates, proteins, and fats — the macronutrients — in giving our bodies energy, structure, and function. CICO, the principle of calories in, calories out, makes it evident that there is no way to avoid taking in fewer calories than you burn each day if you want to lose weight.

➢ The extra importance of protein for weightlifters and exercise enthusiasts in middle age is explained, and there is a list of recommended sources of healthy protein from both animal and plant sources.

> ➤ Different popular diets were covered, and you are encouraged to follow a diet like the Mediterranean, which encourages a wide assortment of fruit and vegetables, lean meat and fish, grains, beans and cereals, nuts and seeds, olive oil, and even red wine, in moderation.

> ➤ Those who follow this diet eat for pleasure as well as for health and fitness and maintain a physically active lifestyle.

Misconceptions about fitness. We concluded with some of the popular misconceptions about weightlifting and exercising at age 40-plus and provided reassurance that *yes, you can*, and *yes, you should* stay healthier, stronger, less likely to suffer injuries, and help resist diseases. You actually do have the time to exercise, despite a busy schedule, you can, and should, lift heavy weights. Both diet and exercise are needed for maintaining a healthy weight, and yes, you can burn fat at your age.

Let's go. If you have not yet started your strengthening and fitness program, what are you waiting for? I would sum up by telling you:

> ➤ "The best time to start was yesterday. The second-best time is now."

Reference List

Alexander, H. (2020, June). What are macronutrients? MD Anderson Cancer Center.

https://www.mdanderson.org/publications/focused-on-health/what-aremacronutrients-.h15-1593780.html

Barrell, A. (2020, Dec. 3). Should you workout when you're sore? Medical News Today.

https://www.medicalnewstoday.com/articles/326892?utm_source=Sailthru%20Email

&utm_medium=Email&utm_campaign=MNT%20Daily%20News&utm_content=20

20-12-18&utm_country=&utm_hcp=&apid=25264436&utm_term=B

Brown, R. (2016, Sept. 16). Top 5 fitness myths of adults over 50. Next Avenue.

https://www.nextavenue.org/top-5-fitness-myths-among-adults-over-50/

Cassetty, S. (2020, Sept. 11). The CICO diet: how it does and does not work for weight loss. Today.

https://www.today.com/health/what-cico-diet-all-about-calories-calories-outdiet-t191457

Cathe. (2019, April 11). What impact does exercise have on blood lipids?

https://cathe.com/what-impact-does-exercise-have-on-blood-lipids/

Current Biology. (2016). Constrained total energy expenditure and metabolic adaptation to physical activity in adult humans.

https://www.cell.com/currentbiology/fulltext/S0960-9822(15)01577-8

da Silva, J., Vinagre, C. et al. (2011, Sept. 9). Resistance training changes LDL metabolism in normolipidemic subjects: a study with a nanoemulsion mimetic of LDL. Atherosclerosis.

https://www.atherosclerosis-journal.com/article/S0021-9150(11)00818-5/abstract

Davis, N. (2019, March 25). Try this: 17 exercises to relieve upper back pain, neck pain, and more. Healthline. https://www.healthline.com/health/fitness-exercise/upper-backpainexercises?slot_pos=article_2&utm_source=Sailthru%20Email&utm_medium=Email& utm_campaign=generalhealth&utm_content=2020-12-01&apid=25264436&rvid=0fcaeb66b8efed5fc78f73c81ad f7036378bf5e4be033e89cfcf a2700293b230

Eliza. (2019, Sept. 16). 5 fitness over 40 myths debunked. Eliza Tips.

https://elizadoalot.com/5-fitness-over-40-myths-debunked/

Frontera, W., Hughes, V., et al. (2000, April). Aging of skeletal muscle: a 12-yr longitudinal study. Journal of Applied Physiology. https://pubmed.ncbi.nlm.nih.gov/10749826/

Gunnars, K. (2019, March 8). 10 science-backed reasons to eat more protein. Healthline.

https://www.healthline.com/nutrition/10-reasons-to-eat-more-protein

Harvard Health Publishing. (2016, February). Preserve your muscle mass.

https://www.health.harvard.edu/staying-healthy/preserve-your-muscle-mass/

Ho, S., Dhaliwal, S., et al. (2012, Aug. 28). The effect of 12 weeks of aerobic, resistance or combination exercise training on cardiovascular risk factors in the overweight and obese in a randomized trial. BMC Public Health.

https://www.ncbi.nlm.nih.gov/pmc/articles/PMC3487794/

Karen. (2019, Sept. 27). Get fit over 40 by rejecting 5 fitness myths. Well Balanced Women.

https://wellbalancedwomen.com/5-fitness-myths-women-over-40/

Mayo Clinic Staff. (2020). Exercise: a drug-free approach to lowering high blood pressure.

https://www.mayoclinic.org/diseases-conditions/high-blood-pressure/in-depth/highblood-pressure/art-20045206

Mayo Clinic Staff. (2020). Exercise and chronic disease: get the facts.

https://www.mayoclinic.org/healthy-lifestyle/fitness/in-depth/exercise-and-chronicdisease/art-20046049

Mayo Clinic Staff. (2020). Nutrition and healthy eating. Paleo diet: what is it and why is it so popular?

https://www.mayoclinic.org/healthy-lifestyle/nutrition-and-healthyeating/in-depth/paleo-diet/art-20111182

National Heart, Lung, and Blood Institute. (2020). Calculate your body mass index.

https://www.nhlbi.nih.gov/health/educational/lose_wt/BMI/bmicalc.htm

National Osteoporosis Foundation. (2020). Osteoporosis exercises for strong bones.

https://www.nof.org/patients/treatment/exercisesafe-movement/osteoporosisexercise-for-strong-bones/

Raman, R. (2017, Sept. 24). Why your metabolism slows down with age. Healthline.

https://www.healthline.com/nutrition/metabolism-and-age

Siddique, H. (2016, Jan. 28). Exercise alone won't cause weight loss, study shows. The Guardian.

https://www.theguardian.com/science/2016/jan/28/study-reveals-thatexercise-alone-wont-cause-weight-loss

Story, C. (2019, Jan. 9). Lowering your high cholesterol: 6 exercises that will pay off. Healthline.

https://www.healthline.com/health/high-cholesterol/treating-with-statins/bestexercises

Tinsley, G. (2018, Jan. 21). 26 foods that help you build lean muscle. Healthline.

https://www.healthline.com/nutrition/26-muscle-building-foods

Tzankoff, S., Norris, A. (1977, Dec. 1). Effects of muscle mass decrease on age-related BMR changes. Journal of Applied Physiology. https://journals.physiology.org/doi/pdf/10.1152/jappl.1977.43.6.1001

U.S. News & World Report. (2021). Keto diet.

https://health.usnews.com/best-diet/keto-diet

Van Pelt, R., Pones, P., et al. (1997, October). Regular exercise and the age-related decline in resting metabolic rate in women. Journal of Clinical Endocrinol Metabolism.

https://pubmed.ncbi.nlm.nih.gov/9329340/

WebMD. (2020). 6 Exercises to help your knees. https://www.webmd.com/painmanagement/knee-pain/injury-knee-pain-16/slideshow-kneeexercises?ecd=wnl_spr_122020&ctr=wnl-spr-122020_nsl-

Bodymodule_Position3&mb=MukfT6opS3AxbF5kSEwI0ng0WleHxvIqssh%40W36l 9r4%3d

Reference List for Images

Fig 1. Herman, Scott. (2010, March 27). How to: dumbbell incline chest press. YouTube.

https://www.youtube.com/watch?v=8iPEnn-ltC8

Fig 2. Herman, Scott. (2010, April 10). How to: seated low row. YouTube.

https://www.youtube.com/watch?v=GZbfZ033f74

Fig 3. IntoSport. (2019, Dec. 8). Dumbbell split squat - fitness gym training. YouTube.

https://www.youtube.com/watch?v=MEG6blZtUpc

Fig 4. Herman, Scott. (2012, Dec. 29). How to: dumbbell bent-over row. YouTube.

https://www.youtube.com/watch?v=6TSP1TRMUzs

Fig 5. Calabrese, A. (2014, Sept. 1). How to upright row - proper form and tips. YouTube.

https://www.youtube.com/watch?v=VIoihl5ZZzM

Fig 6. Azar, B. (2012, Aug. 21). How to do a barbell curl/arm workout. Howcast/YouTube.

https://www.youtube.com/watch?v=kwG2ipFRgfo

Fig 7. Herman, S. (2010, Fe. 1). How to: dumbbell lateral side raise. YouTube.

https://www.youtube.com/watch?v=3VcKaXpzqRo

Fig 8. Henson, J. (2015, June 18). How to do a proper plank. Body Mind Wellness Clinic/YouTube.

https://www.youtube.com/watch?v=gvHVdNVBu6s

Fig 9. McKee, K. (2015, Dec. 11). How to do a body-weight squat. Health Magazine/YouTube.

https://www.youtube.com/watch?v=LyidZ42Iy9Q

Fig 10. Syuki, R. (2020, May 30). How to do lying leg raises for abs. YouTube.

https://www.youtube.com/watch?v=UvcTNVbjTYo

Fig 11. Rilinger, H. (2015, Aug. 25). How to do a push-up. Dr. Oz/YouTube.

https://www.youtube.com/watch?v=rjc0O7OXS3g

Fig 12. Crossfit. (2019, Feb. 1). The strict pull-up. YouTube.

https://www.youtube.com/watch?v=HRV5YKKaeVw

Fig 13. Critical Bench. (2018, Sep. 24). Hanging leg raise done right. YouTube.

https://www.youtube.com/watch?v=lS5B0MmLgZs

Fig 14. Herman, S. (2011, Oct. 1). How to: bench dips. YouTube.
Fig https://www.youtube.com/watch?v=c3ZGl4pAwZ4

BOOK 3

Baz Thompson

Building Muscle

for Beginners

The Complete Blueprint to Building Muscle with Weight Lifting

Introduction

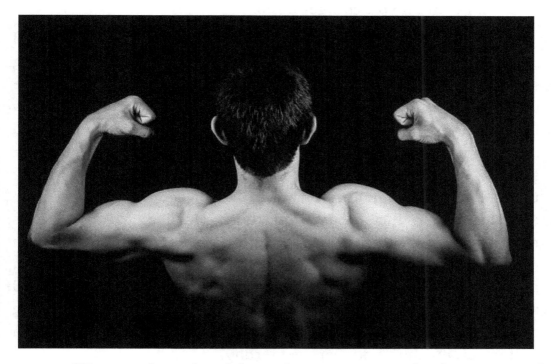

"No man has the right to be an amateur in the matter of physical training. It is a shame for a man to grow old without seeing the beauty and strength of which his body is capable." - Socrates.

Who would have known that one of history's greatest thinkers would have the same kind of passion for physical training that he did for philosophy and contemplation? You can't deny that he has a very strong argument here. As human beings, our very existence is a miracle in itself. Think of how many conceivable determinants needed to be satisfied in order for you to get here - to be who you are right at this very moment. The sheer mathematics of it is almost incomprehensible. It would be an awful waste of your life if you didn't push yourself to find out just how far you can go; to discover how much you can endure; to see how much you can get done.

If you're someone who aspires to have a chiseled and muscular frame, then that's a good thing. There is nothing shallow or pretentious about you wanting to look good and have a better build. Whenever someone tells you that it's really shallow for you to obsess over building your body, just tell them that you have Socrates on your side and that man was far from being shallow. You understand this journey that you wish to embark upon. It's more than just trying to get bigger biceps or a more sculpted chest. It's about what these physical manifestations represent. It's about the hard work and the commitment that you put into getting what you want. By picking up this book, you prove to yourself and the world that you have a curious soul and are eager to learn. You are showing that you aren't afraid of going after what you want. That's always the first step to becoming a better person than you were yesterday.

Of course, having the motivation to do good and make something of yourself is not enough. You also need the know-how and the proper game plan necessary to get you from where you are now to where you want to be. That's precisely what this book is going to help you out with. Whenever you look at the world's elite athletes and see their prime bodies that look like the gods themselves have sculpted them, it can be very easy to become discouraged and think that you would never be able to amount to that. However, you have to understand that all of these elite athletes started out somewhere. In fact, a lot of them may have started out in worse conditions than the current shape that you're in right now. The only thing that separates you from them is the amount of work that they've already put in. Fortunately for you, there is still time left for you to do everything that it takes to get your desired body. This book will help shed light on the art of bodybuilding and all of the science that goes into it. It's imperative that you gain a fundamental academic understanding of how your body works and what you need to do to take care of it. This book will also go into detail into the roles of exercise and nutrition and how you can use these tools to sculpt your dream physical form. Most importantly, this book is going to present to you all of the basic knowledge that you need to design your own path moving forward.

At the end of the day, everyone's bodies are all shaped differently. This is why you must be able to develop a plan for yourself to make sure that it's tailor-fitted to your own personal needs and goals. Don't worry. It's not as complicated as it seems. This book is going to help walk you through the entire process in a very structured and purposeful manner, so you can avoid any misunderstandings about what to do in order for you to achieve your goals.

However, aside from talking about what this book is, it's also important to emphasize what this book isn't going to be. First of all, this book isn't going to do the work for you. Just reading this book alone doesn't guarantee that you're automatically going to get the body that you want. The most crucial step here is for you to apply your knowledge to your everyday life to the best of your ability. This book will not serve as a magic pill that is a one-size-fits-all solution to all of your problems. Understand that all human beings are different. The training plan for an elite athlete is not always going to be effective for a novice or beginner. However, what this book can do is provide you with enough knowledge and perspective to understand the potential and limitations of your own body. It doesn't matter whether you're overweight, differently-abled, or whatever. It doesn't matter if you're allergic to gluten or if you have diabetes. All of the principles that will be presented in this book can still help you out in your fitness journey.

Benefits of Lean and Healthy Muscle

Building

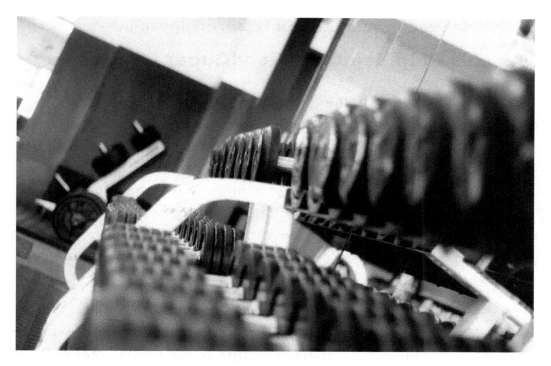

To provide you with more incentive to pursue your goals of getting bigger, better-defined muscles, you should know that the benefits of your hard work exceed mere aesthetics. It's not just about how your body is going to look on the outside. Sure, it can make you feel great to know that you look good. But a lot of the benefits can also be found on the inside. Sure, if you ask many diehard bodybuilders, they will tell you that they derive a lot of joy and fulfillment from being able to achieve their goals. The fulfillment that you get is a benefit in itself, but it's also so much more than that. Sure, weight training is very much concerned with the actual building of a muscle, but there are other physical benefits to strength training as well. This is a common misconception that many have about people who look to build muscle.

Here are just a few of the many ways in which building muscle can lead to you having a better quality of life:

Muscles Help Regulate Blood Sugar Levels

Muscles in themselves don't necessarily regulate the body's blood sugar levels per se. Rather, it's the resistance training that is required for bodybuilding that helps regulate the body's blood sugar levels. In fact, many doctors recommend resistance or anaerobic training for anyone who might have Type 2 Diabetes. This is because strength training helps improve your body's ability to process glucose and deliver it to the muscle, thus decreasing your body's blood sugar levels at any given moment.

Muscles Help Control Body Fat

Muscles are known to help control the body fat levels in your body because they increase your metabolism. Metabolism is essentially the process of converting your body's stored fat into energy for movement and bodily functions. So, the more muscles you have, the more energy that is required for your body to function. The more energy you burn, the more fat that you lose as well. Bulking up isn't just about getting sculpted. It's also about getting rid of that stubborn fat which is proven to be a leading cause for disease in many people.

Muscles Give You More Functional Strength

Getting bigger and stronger as a result of resistance training doesn't just mean that you get to lift heavier weights at the gym. All of this added strength and functionality can apply to your everyday life as well. When you are a stronger person, life just generally becomes easier for you. It won't be a problem having to lift heavy boxes when you move. You won't have to worry about pulling yourself up onto something. The exercises that you do at the gym translate to better efficiency in movement for everyday life. However, this might also mean that your friends will be calling you first when they need help lifting something heavy.

Muscles Reduce the Risk of Cancer and Cardiovascular Disease

Earlier, it was mentioned that muscles help control the level of fat in your body. However, not all fats are created equal. There is such a thing as visceral fat which can be very harmful to your health. Visceral fat is a kind of fat that attaches itself on top of your major organs. All of this added fat can put unnecessary stress on your organs and potentially cause them to malfunction. This means that your major organs like your heart, liver, or kidneys can be compromised and cause some serious illnesses for you. On top of that, visceral fat is also notorious for enabling the development of cancerous tissues. By engaging in regular strength training, you are minimizing the likelihood of developing harmful visceral fat.

Muscles Strengthen Bones, Ligaments, and Joints

Having bigger and stronger muscles will also help make you a more durable person overall. This is especially useful if you're an athlete who always likes to stay active. For example, if you are a long-distance runner, you can still stand to benefit from doing some bodybuilding and strength training every once in a while. Adding more muscle to your frame will help lessen the stress and impact on your joints and bones. Imagine every single step that you take while running and the amount of stress that can have on your knees. If you have stronger leg muscles, they can help take some of the tension away from your joints by absorbing most of the impact.

Muscle-Building Improves Your Emotional and Mental Health

Again, muscles in themselves might not necessarily be primarily responsible for improving your mental and emotional health, but resistance training can help support a healthier state of mind. Whenever you exercise, your brain triggers the release of hormones called endorphins. These are also often referred to as the happy hormones. They are responsible for making you feel like you've accomplished something and they put you in a good mood. They are often described as being able to provide people with a natural high.

Muscles Lengthen Your Lifespan

Lastly, having a lean mean fighting machine as a body is also likely to lengthen your lifespan. For one, we've already talked about how you are less likely to contract certain harmful diseases and illnesses if you have lower body fat and higher muscle mass. That fact alone can really improve your chances of living a longer life. However, having an improved state of mental and emotional health as a result of consistent exercise can also help you live longer. This mental and emotional boost can help you relieve stress, which is known to be one of the biggest killers in the medical world. With consistent exercise, you are also effectively making yourself more invulnerable to stress.

And there you have it. Those are just some of the most important benefits that you can get from devoting more time and effort to sculpting your body. Of course, by now, you're probably raring to go, but you've got to tone it down a little bit. Remember that you need a game plan first. You need to take a structured and methodical approach to develop your physical fitness. The first step to doing so is understanding how your body works and the science that goes into biomechanics, metabolism, catabolism, and other concepts involved in muscle building.

Chapter 1

An Introduction to Building Muscle

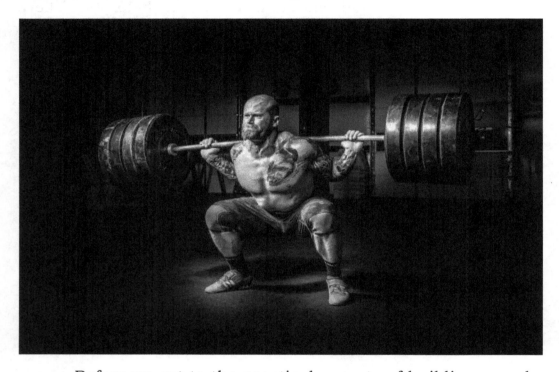

Before we get to the practical aspects of building muscle, we have to discuss the biological first. Don't worry. This isn't going to be some super complex scientific discussion on physiology and biomechanics. You don't need to be a medical doctor or have a specialization in biology for you to understand everything that's going to be discussed here. We are going to keep things as simple as can be. Again, this is a book that is designed for anyone to read and be able to understand. You won't have to worry about encountering ideas or concepts that you wouldn't be able to comprehend or apply to your own life.

In this chapter, we are going to delve deeper into what exactly happens in your body whenever you work out and try to build muscle. Whenever you do a bicep curl, your muscles don't just magically grow ever so slightly with every rep. That's not how the muscle building process works. It's a lot more complex than that. By the time you finish this chapter, you will gain a more profound understanding of how your muscles gain mass and what you can do to stimulate that process.

Consider the knowledge in this introductory chapter as a prerequisite to everything that you'll learn in the rest of the book. This will be the foundation for all of the knowledge that you will absorb and is crucial to your journey towards getting the body of your dreams. This chapter is going to tackle concepts like clean and dirty bulking, hypertrophy, rest and recovery, range of motion, strength imbalance, and more. With this chapter, we are laying the groundwork and the blueprint for the future version of yourself.

How do Muscles Grow? The Science of Hypertrophy

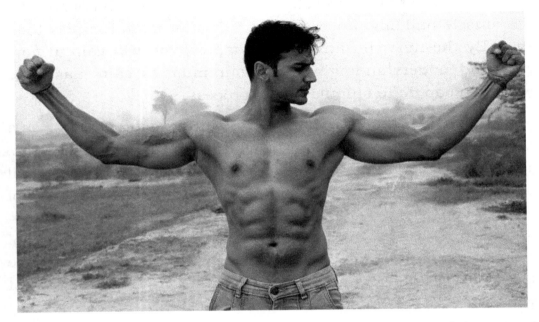

You know that going to the gym, lifting weights, and eating protein can help you bulk up and get bigger. You probably know this because of your exposure to popular media or you might have some friends who are avid gym rats. And yes, these activities can definitely contribute to muscle growth. But how? That's what we're going to try to explain in the simplest terms possible right now. The actual process of building muscle is called hypertrophy. Scientifically, this is the process of the increase and growth of muscle cells in your body. Now, there are two types of hypertrophy that you need to know about, especially when you're planning out your strength and training program. First, there is myofibrillar hypertrophy. This deals with the increase in the size of your body parts that are involved in muscle contraction. Then, there is sarcoplasmic hypertrophy. This is the increase in your muscle's ability to store glycogen. To the layman, these two classifications of hypertrophy might not necessarily be all that important. However, if you're really going to drill down on your training, you need to pay more attention. Myofibrillar hypertrophy has to do with improving your muscle's capacity for strength and speed. This means that your movements are more explosive when you do this kind of muscle building. On the other hand, sarcoplasmic hypertrophy has more to do with sustained efforts and endurance. This kind of training allows you to keep moving over long periods of time.

Now, it still begs the question, how exactly does hypertrophy work? Well, it's all a matter of breaking to build. You have to break your muscle fibers down to allow for space for new fibers to grow and add to your mass. It's that simple. Whenever you perform a movement that stresses your muscle fibers at a certain frequency, your muscle fibers will break and become damaged. This is the reason you might feel sore for a day or two after a session of heavy lifting. The soreness that you feel is the damaged muscle fibers in your body. Now, that these fibers are broken, you need to replace them in order to maximize the recovery process by loading up on protein. Proteins are made up of amino acids which play a crucial role in the building of muscle and spearheading the body's recovery. When you consume protein, these molecules enter your bloodstream and travel to the areas of your body where your muscle fibers are broken. Then, they will fill the gaps and add to your body's overall mass.

This might all seem theoretical to you, so let's try to paint a clearer picture of what is taking place in your body when you're trying to build muscle. Imagine yourself performing a few reps of the bench press. This is a movement that requires the effort of your pectoral muscles, triceps, and front shoulders. The more reps that you perform at a challenging weight, the more you are essentially stressing these muscles out to the point of mechanical damage and metabolic fatigue. This means that your muscles are breaking down and are losing the energy that they need to sustain this movement for a longer period of time. This is why the reps on the bench press become increasingly more difficult the more reps you complete.

Over time, as the muscles become bigger and stronger, certain movements become easier to perform. This is why the concept of progressive overload is important in building muscle. If we go back to the bench press example, imagine that you start out performing five sets of five reps of the bench press at 135 lbs. three times a week. After the first couple of sessions, it might feel very challenging for you. But then, it gets easier every time. This is because your muscles are growing and learning to adapt to the movement. If you continue to stick to this workout scheme, your muscles will be less likely to break and engage in hypertrophy. This is why it's advisable to increase either the intensity or the volume of your workouts gradually over time. So, after a couple of weeks of lifting 135 lbs with a 5x5 rep scheme, you can try increasing the load or the number of reps. Maybe you can do 145 lbs with the same rep scheme or you can keep the load and add another set to every session. This way, you are constantly stimulating your muscles and challenging them to the point of fibral breakage.

Approaches to Hypertrophy

The Role of Calories in Building Muscle

Now, we've talked about how hypertrophy is essentially a process of breaking to build. You break your muscle fibers down in order to build them up. While there is no other natural way to build muscle other than through hypertrophy, there are still many approaches to the break to build method. In particular, there are two main methods that we will be focusing on in this book. There is the slow and lean bulk and the overloaded dirty bulk. Before we can discuss the differences between these two methods of bulking up, you have to orient yourself on the roles that calories play.

When you think of calories in the fitness industry, you might get the impression that these are substances that you need to stay away from because they will make you fat. However, what most people don't realize is that calories in themselves are not fattening. All food contains a certain amount of calories and these calories are made up of vital nutrients that your body needs to sustain itself. Earlier, we discussed how protein is a crucial ingredient to the process of hypertrophy. Every gram of protein that you consume carries around four calories. Without any calories, your body would not be able to sustain itself. You wouldn't be able to survive.

Every single second you're alive, your body is continually using up calories whether you realize it or not. Sure, you might know that performing strenuous movements like running, jumping, and heavy lifting can burn a significant amount of calories. But what you may not know is that you're still burning calories even when you're just lying down. You're even burning calories as you sleep. This is because your calories are converted into glucose which is used as fuel for your body to function properly. Every time your heart beats, it requires energy. Every time your lungs contract and expand, they require energy. Whenever your intestines process and break down your food, they require calories. This means that the food that you eat gets converted into the energy that is responsible for allowing your organs to function properly.

However, calories often get demonized in the fitness industry because many people often overindulge in their food to the point where they are consuming more calories than they are burning up. We all have different caloric requirements depending on how our bodies are made up and the kinds of activities that we do every day. A person with a larger build who works as a hauler for a living will require more daily calories than a slender individual who has a desk job. Now, in terms of training for building muscle, you will require a specific number of calories in order for you to sustain your daily output. If you're not eating enough calories, especially from protein, then you are compromising the entire hypertrophic process. This is because you are not feeding your muscles enough protein to facilitate the building process.

We will go into more detail about calories and general nutrition later on in the book. This is a topic that will require its own chapter and there are many more details that need to be addressed.

Clean Bulk vs Dirty Bulk

When you structure your diet and training scheme, there are two things that you need to familiarize yourself with: caloric deficits and caloric surpluses. You get into a caloric deficit when you consume fewer calories than your body requires to function daily. This can also mean longer recovery times for sore and broken down muscle fibers. You get a caloric surplus when you consume more calories than you are using. This ensures that your body is getting the calories that it needs to function, but if done excessively, it can also lead to weight gain and the development of fatty tissues.

Given that, there are typically two approaches that bodybuilders will take when it comes to building muscle: clean bulking and dirty bulking. A clean bulk is when someone does strenuous strength training and eats just about the right amount of calories that hovers over the line in terms of how much they're burning off every day. So, if you calculate that you're burning off around 3000-3500 calories per day, then that would also be the number of calories you consume when you're on a clean bulk. The pros of this method include you making sure that you are never eating excessively. You are still engaging in hypertrophy while minimizing the development of fat. However, with this kind of dieting method, it's also possible that you aren't eating as much as you should be. Calorie counting is not an exact science. This is why progress might seem very slow and minimal with this kind of approach to hypertrophy.

Then, there is the dirty bulk. This is when you engage in intense strength and resistance training and you eat substantially more calories than you know that you're burning every day. Clean bulking involves you toeing the line of your caloric output every day. Dirty bulking has you going over that line consistently. This might be beneficial to some people who are looking for clearer and more immediate results with their hypertrophy. However, it also leaves most others prone to unnecessary fat gain.

Should You Do Cardio While Building Muscle?

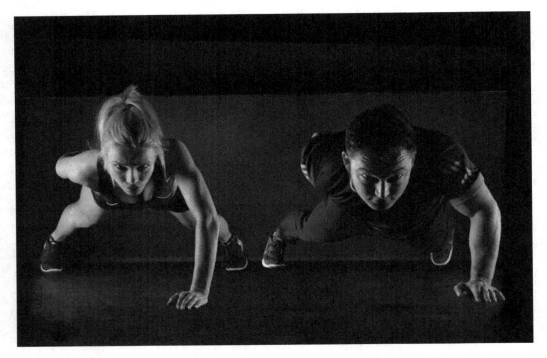

To this day, the fitness community remains divided on the matter and there's a reason for that. There is no direct answer that just applies to everyone. Again, it's always going to be a case by case basis depending on a person's physiological makeup and goals. Don't worry. This is not a cop-out. In general, the answer to "Should you do cardio while building muscle?" is always going to be yes. Cardiovascular exercises are good for the heart and they can benefit everyone. However, that isn't the right question to ask. Rather, the right question lies in how much cardio should you be doing when you're trying to build muscle. But in order to answer that question, there are two other questions that you need to address first.

What is your body type and what are your goals?

Addressing Your Body Type

Are you a naturally skinny person who seems to always stay lean no matter how much you eat? Do you already have a big build but it's made up mostly of flab? Are you the kind of person who seems to gain muscle relatively easily? These are all questions that you need to ask yourself in order to determine your body type. We will delve deeper into the science of body types in the next chapter. But for now, what you need to know is that the more fat you already have in your body, then the more cardio that you need to do. Of course, building muscle through strength and resistance training can also help facilitate fat loss. However, you can supplement your fat loss efforts by doing more cardiovascular activities like running or jumping ropes.

Catering to Your Goals

Another important detail that you need to take into consideration is what goals you have for yourself. As a general rule of thumb, the leaner and more defined you want your muscles to appear, you might have to do a little more cardio than the typical bodybuilder. However, if you're someone who is focusing more on bulk and you don't care so much about definition, then you shouldn't really concern yourself too much with cardio at all.

Bottom Line

This is why the fitness community continues to be so divided when trying to answer this question. No one answer is suitable for all bodybuilders. It's all subject to your own personal interpretation of your situation and your goals. Ultimately, the best that you can do is analyze the most ideal theoretical framework to follow and adopt it for yourself. If you get the results that you want, then that's great. If you don't feel like you're progressing over time, then don't be afraid to go back to the drawing board.

The Importance of Sleep and Recovery

We won't delve too much into this concept for this initial chapter because it's far too complex and it requires a full chapter on its own. However, it's still essential to stress the importance of incorporating sleep and recovery into planning for your muscle building process. There are plenty of people who will come up with the most detailed diet plans and the most comprehensive training programs for you to follow and that's a good thing. But it's also important that you develop a good sleep and recovery plan for yourself as well. Good sleep is what enables you to have the energy every day to sustain your strenuous workouts. Your recovery time is also important as this is where the "build" aspect of the break to build process takes place.

The time you spend at the gym training is you breaking your muscles. The time you spend recovering is your body building itself up. Again, this is something that you will be briefed on more comprehensively in a later chapter. But for now, it's important that you know that sleep and recovery are integral aspects of the muscle building process.

Chapter 2

Understanding Your Body Type

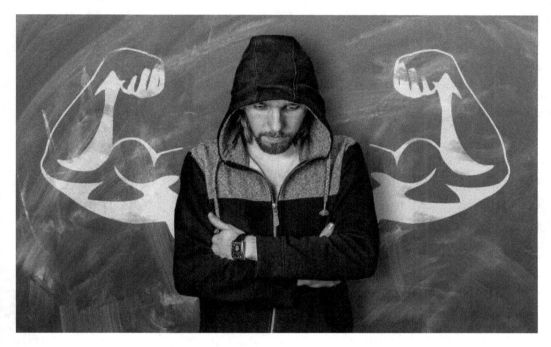

Not everyone is going to be wired the same way. This is why the concept of bodybuilding is a lot more complex than most people make it out to be. A training program that proves effective for one person isn't necessarily going to be one that works for another. You and a friend might share the same personal trainer and the same training routine, but you might not necessarily get the same results. You might be doing all of the same things, but your bodies might be responding differently.

This chapter will give you more insight into the different body types and how they are different.

It's important that you really understand your body type because it is the most important tool for achieving optimal fitness. The most important tool is not a barbell. It's not a dumbbell. It's not a squat rack. It's your body. This is why you need to take some time to really understand your body's ins and outs to determine your body type. Once you are familiar with your body type, then you will be in a better position to plot your point of attack for your fitness goals and objectives.

The Three Main Body Types

There are three distinct body types that most people typically tend to fall under, in bodybuilding. These body types can have a dramatic impact on how your body responds to training stimuli, nutrition, recovery, and other factors that are involved in building muscle. Given that, gaining knowledge of the ins and outs of your body type will allow you to understand what you need to do in order for you to find success. It was mentioned that there are three distinct body types that we will be discussing here, however, it's important to note that you're not necessarily just bound to one category all of the time. Sometimes, people can start out as one type when they are younger and then gradually transition to another body type as they get older. There are a variety of factors that go into determining your body type, such as genetics, lifestyle, physical activity, health history, and more. With that reminder out of the way, let's get right into discussing the differences between being an ectomorph, endomorph, and mesomorph.

Ectomorph

The first body type to be discussed here is the ectomorph. This is the type of person who struggles to gain weight despite feeling full whenever they eat. The ectomorph struggles to gain fat or muscle and is often referred to as hard gainers. When trying to build muscles, ectomorphs will have to consume a lot more lean protein (sometimes, with the help of supplements) in order to see results. Also, ectomorphs tend to progress more slowly when it comes to building strength as compared to the other body types. Whenever they don't eat enough, they are also prone to losing weight a lot more quickly than others.

The main reason that ectomorphs struggle with weight gain is because of their fast metabolism. They have bodies that are so efficient at processing carbohydrates and converting them into fuel for energy that none of these get left behind in the body as stored fats. As much as possible, ectomorphs need to limit cardiovascular activity so as not to lose any unnecessary calories that might compromise the muscle building process.

What Does an Ectomorph Look Like?

Typically, an ectomorph who doesn't work out or doesn't do any kind of resistance training will have the build of the stereotypical marathon runner. They might have visible abs as the result of not having any fat around the belly rather than from core exercises. Sometimes, ectomorphs can still have a little fat around the body, but the fat will still be contained in a relatively small frame.

The Dos and Don'ts of an Ectomorph

The first thing that you need to remember as an ectomorph is that you need to stay away from the treadmill as much as possible. There's no need for you to be doing cardio. In a bodybuilding program, cardio is typically used as a tool for burning fat in order to highlight the definitions of muscles. However, since you're an ectomorph, your body is already doing a good enough job of burning fat on its own. If you do cardio, you risk burning more calories than you would typically want and your muscles end up getting broken down and converted into energy as compensation.

Ideally, you will want to perform compound movements for a huge bulk of your training regimen. These are movements designed to recruit different muscle groups to accurately and safely perform a given task. Also, look for high volumes in terms of rep schemes. This is the best way for you to progressively build your strength given your body type.

Lastly, you want to make sure that you have a high calorie diet. Again, your body type is one that enables the fast processing of food and the burning of calories. This means you have to constantly replenish your energy stores so that your body doesn't end up breaking your muscles. Go for a lot of healthy complex carbs and lean protein to help you bulk up. Healthy fat from olive oil or nuts is also good for helping your body process nutrients more efficiently. Fats also carry more calories per gram relative to the two other macronutrients. Also, don't be afraid to make use of supplements to make sure that you are getting all of the nutrients that you need to sustain your workouts.

Endomorph

An endomorph is someone who is very good at retaining fuel storage. They tend to have higher amounts of fat and muscles concentrated on the lower extremities of the body. Many trainers and experts will say that endomorphs have the most difficult time in terms of managing weight and developing overall fitness. If you are an endomorph, gaining weight is going to be a relatively easy process for you. Conversely, losing weight and cutting fat is going to be more difficult for you than it is for others. You will have a tendency to have a wider torso and legs. It's very easy for you to build muscle, but it's hard for you to gain LEAN muscle. That means that while you may be building your muscles through caloric surpluses, it's also likely that you're getting fatter at the same time.

Of course, this isn't to say that getting a lean and trim body is totally impossible for you. There are many endomorphs out there who have chiseled physiques as the result of their hard work and strict commitment to their fitness regimens. You just have to make sure that you really put in the hard work at the gym and in the kitchen with your diet. Getting strong is very easy for you, but losing the fat while maintaining that strength might prove to be a challenge.

What Does an Endomorph Look Like?

If you are an endomorph, it's likely that you will have what most people refer to as a stocky or blocky build. You might have a wider rib cage than most and your hips might be just as wide, if not wider than your collarbones. You might also have thicker joints and flabbier limbs than most. Muscle definition is still possible in endomorphs, but they are likely to be accompanied by lumps of fat as well. The most prominent endomorphs in the sporting world tend to be American football players, sumo wrestlers, and Olympic weightlifters.

The Dos and Don'ts of an Endomorph

The first thing you could be doing wrong as an endomorph is spending hours at a time on a treadmill or elliptical machine. Sure, it might seem like a good idea to devote more time to cardio work since you aren't necessarily built lean, but, this wouldn't be an efficient use of your time, especially if you're looking to build muscle. Rather than doing slow steady-state cardiovascular work, try using bursts or intervals of high-intensity training instead. You get all of the benefits of the fat burn while you're exercising, and you get to rev up your metabolism for when you're at rest as well. For example, instead of running at a steady pace on a treadmill for 30 minutes, try doing a 15-minute interval of 30-second sprints and 30-second walks.

Another thing that you should do is lift heavier loads. You might believe that, since you're on the stockier side, you need to focus on shedding fat before building muscle. However, you can use muscle building as a tool for you to burn fat more effectively. The best way to do this is to lift heavy weights at low to moderate reps with minimal recovery periods in between sets.

In terms of your diet, limit your carbohydrate intake as much as possible. This will force your body to turn to your stored fats as a source of fuel. Also, load up on a lot of lean protein and fiber. This is just to make sure that while your body is burning stored fat for fuel, your muscles are constantly being fed. This means you need to stay away from food like bread and rice. Focus more on green vegetables as a source of carbohydrates.

Mesomorph

When it comes to body types for bodybuilding, you must consider yourself blessed if you are a mesomorph. You have the type of body that is most primed for building lean muscle without gaining too much fat. It's relatively easier for you to get that athletic build that you want than it would be for an endomorph who leans towards being stocky and an ectomorph who is skinny. There are plenty of people around the world who look like they are athletes despite having poor nutrition and exercise regimens. These are the ones who are likely to be considered as mesomorphs.

However, it's important to remember that body types aren't always set in stone. Just because you might be a mesomorph in your teens and early twenties doesn't mean that you're going to stay that way. A lot of the time, as you get older, your metabolism slows down and it'll be harder for you to keep the fat away. This is why it's still important for mesomorphs to incorporate healthy training and nutrition habits into their daily lives if they are to remain healthy and fit. Being a mesomorph puts you at a physiological advantage when competing against the other two body types. But that doesn't mean that you shouldn't be putting in the time and hard work necessary for you to get the real body you want.

What Does a Mesomorph Look Like?

Ultimately, a mesomorph is someone who looks like they spend a considerable amount of time at the gym even when that isn't the case. Also, mesomorphs are those who tend to pack on muscle relatively quickly. They also find it a lot easier to gain strength and explosiveness in a relatively short amount of time. Like an endomorph, you are likely to have wide shoulders and a strong-looking chest. However, you're going to be a lot trimmer around the waste as compared to the endomorph. You are less likely to develop belly fat.

You are also more inclined to develop sculpted legs, particularly with the quadriceps and calves.

The Dos and Don'ts of a Mesomorph

Again, since mesomorphs are typically blessed with good genetics, there is a high chance that they will become complacent with their diet and training. This might not necessarily be a problem at the start. However, over a sustained period of time, this can prove to be very harmful. This is why mesomorphs need to establish more measurable and tangible goals for themselves. This way, they stay more motivated to workout as they chase real targets.

Also, incorporate regular progression in your workouts as much as possible. Again, you are blessed with good genes and you will likely develop your strength at a far more rapid rate than the other two body types. This means that you need to constantly be upping your workout's difficulty so that your progress never stagnates. If you make your workouts difficult, this means that you are bringing new stimuli every single time you train. Also, try to incorporate more explosive movements into your training routine. Focus on functional movements like box jumps, sprints, pull-ups, and other training tools that translate to function in everyday life.

Final Thoughts

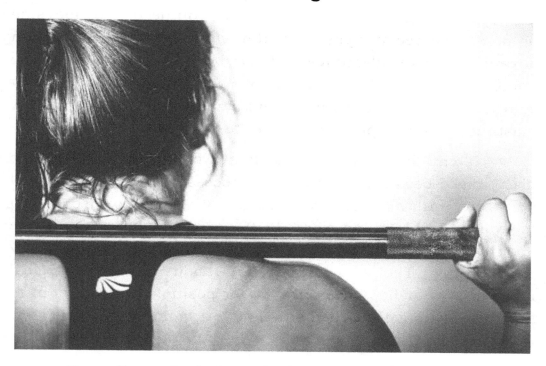

Regardless of whatever body type you fall under, there's no need to feel discouraged because of the genetic makeup of your body. Sure, you might feel like other people will have an advantage because they have a certain body type. But the struggle is all the same. At the end of the day, no one gets their ideal body without putting in the hard work. It doesn't matter whether you're an ectomorph, endomorph, or mesomorph. If you're lazy and unmotivated, you aren't going to get results. Ultimately, it helps to have better tools that will help you to succeed. However, all of these tools are pointless unless you put them to good use.

Having an ideal body type is an advantage. But not having an ideal body type should not be a deterrent either. Keep in mind that the journey that you're about to embark on is yours and yours alone. If other people are progressing faster than you, it's irrelevant. You are the only person that you need to be focusing on here. Just because you know that your body type has certain advantages or disadvantages relative to other people is not the point. The point of this entire chapter is to point out to you how your body responds to certain stimuli so that you can design the most ideal training plan that caters to your specific needs.

It can be so easy to look at your body and become discouraged because you might not necessarily have the natural body type you want. However, that is not a viable excuse for you to avoid putting in the work. In fact, gaining more knowledge about your body type should serve as an incentive for you to try even harder. The smarter you are about the physiological makeup of your body, then the better position you will be in to find success in getting the body that you want.

Chapter 3

Nutrition

Contrary to popular belief, building the perfect body isn't just about what you do in the gym. You can do all of the bicep curls and back squats in the world. But if you have terrible eating habits, you're never really going to maximize your body's potential fully. You can't outrun a bad diet, both literally and figuratively. It's that simple. This is why this portion of the book is going to focus more on the work that you do in the kitchen as opposed to the gym. You will come to realize that everything that goes into your mouth can do a lot more for your body than anything that you can do with a barbell or weights.

You will find that this is a pretty consistent theme in this book, but there isn't really any one way to go about dieting. Different diets can have different effects on different people. You've already gotten a glimpse of that earlier when we talked about the different body types and how these people carry different needs both in training and in nutrition. This chapter isn't necessarily going to advocate for one particular diet over another. Don't expect that. Rather, what you can expect is to gain a more in-depth understanding of fundamental nutrition principles so that you can figure out what kind of diet would suit your body type and training regimen best.

In this chapter, we're going to touch on the basics of macronutrients and why you need to be paying attention to them. We are also going to take a deeper dive into the concept of metabolism and calories, and how you can construct your own metabolic plan based on your lifestyle and body type. You will also be briefed on some examples of healthy food items and meals that you should be incorporating into your diet. Finally, you will be given some concrete tips and tricks that will help you make the most of your diet as you pursue your goal body.

The Role of Nutrition in Building Muscle

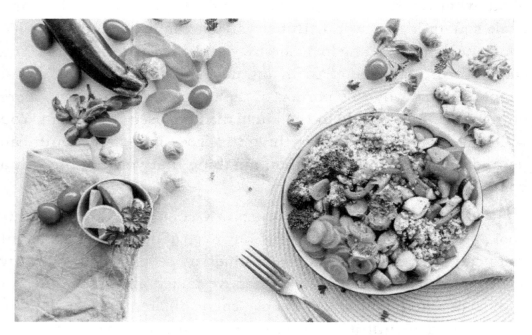

It's time for a hot take: you're wasting your time at the gym if you're just going to eat a lot of crappy food for every meal. You probably already know from your lessons as a kid that you need to have a well-balanced diet in order for you to stay healthy. This is why, as a child, you were always force-fed vegetables even though all you probably wanted to eat were hotdogs and cereal. Hopefully, you've outgrown that phase and have developed a more sophisticated palate. Of course, there are still some adults who might be eating more vegetables now than they did back when they were younger. But how much is the appropriate amount? Should you be eating more meat? Isn't eating meat supposedly bad for you?

Are all fats bad? Then why do some people say that there's such a thing as good fats?

These are all very valid questions that you might have. Nutrition is a messy game and this is why a lot of people become intimidated before starting a new diet. However, the more that you study nutrition and its basic principles, the simpler and clearer everything becomes. This is especially true if you're the kind of person who pays a great deal of attention to how your body looks and how it functions. And if you're reading this book, then there's a good chance that you are indeed that kind of person.

Building the optimal body is not a feat that can be achieved by hard training alone. Again, this is a break to-build process and the training that you do in the gym is merely the breaking aspect of it. The food that you put into your mouth is responsible for building your physique. For one, food is going to help give you the strength and energy to complete your workouts. Also, food is responsible for strengthening your muscles and joints to the point where they increase your build and overall physique.

That is exactly how you should view your relationship with food. You would never be able to perform well at the gym if you're not eating right. Also, you wouldn't be able to grow your muscles if you aren't feeding them properly. The role of nutrition in building muscle is two-fold. It impacts both your performance and your body's overall aesthetics. If you obsess over the amount of weight that you pull and the number of reps that you execute, then you need to do the same with your food as well. You have to obsess over the number of calories that you eat and how much protein you're taking in. These are all little details that can add up over time to a dramatic impact and success for your body.

The Value of Protein

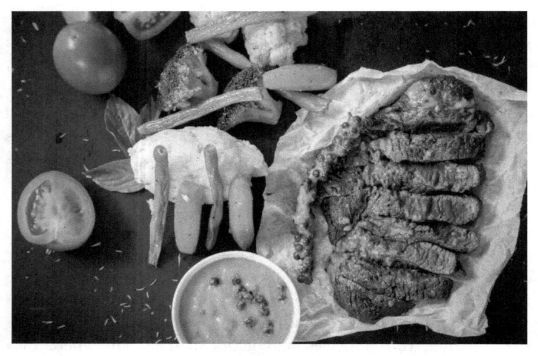

You probably already know by now that bodybuilders and athletes live off protein. But what you may not know if you're a nutrition novice is that protein only comprises one of the three macronutrients that you need to be incorporating into your diet. Yes, protein serves as a very important building block for feeding your muscles and strengthening your joints. However, you can't just live off protein alone. You need to understand the relationship that protein has your body and the other macronutrients as well. This way, you have a more holistic approach to understanding your nutrition and developing a plan for yourself.

Figuring Out the Three Macronutrients

If you recall all the old lessons you had about nutrition, you might remember that every food item might be rich in a particular nutrient. Also, you might recall that every nutrient carries a distinct benefit for your body. For example, you might have been told that carrots were rich in Vitamin A. This meant that you would have improved eyesight. Also, you might have learned that oranges are rich in Vitamin C. This means that they can help you improve your immune system. Now, it's good if you really familiarize yourself with all these nutrients and what food you can source them from. However, for the purposes of building muscle, there are only three nutrients that you need to really pay attention to. They're referred to as the macronutrients and they comprise carbohydrates, fat, and protein.

In this segment on nutrition, you are going to be briefed on the different values of each macronutrient and what roles they play in your quest to build your physique. Again, it's not just about eating as much protein as you can. You don't want to be a meathead. Once you have a better understanding of all three macronutrients, you will be in a better position to have a truly more well-balanced diet... the same one that your grade school teachers and parents tried to teach you about when you were younger.

Carbohydrates

The first macronutrient that you need to know about is carbohydrates or carbs for short. Too often, carbs will get a bad rap in the fitness community because they are closely associated with food like donuts or pizza. Naturally, if you are eating a diet that consists of copious amounts of those particular food items, you're going to get fat. However, while these high-carb food items might be bad for you, carbs in themselves aren't so bad.

In terms of calories, carbs only carry four calories per gram. This is substantially much fewer calories per gram than fat. However, the problem with carbohydrates when it comes to building muscle isn't just about how many calories they have. It more has to do with how your body is processing those calories internally. Carbs serve as readily available sources of fuel for your body. If your body detects carbs in your system, it immediately begins processing those carbs to be converted to glucose. This glucose is what will serve as fuel for you to run, jump, lift, breathe, and anything that requires the recruitment of any part of your body. So, if you're someone who trains in the gym regularly, then you need your carbohydrates to fuel your workouts. Sometimes, you might even get that little extra push during your training sessions as a result of carb consumption. Although, any leftover carbs that aren't processed for energy will be turned into stored fat for future use. It's essentially your body's way of preparing itself in case you need a quick supply of energy in the future but don't have any immediate access to food.

Given that, it's important that you only consume as many carbs as you need at any given time. This way, you are assured that you are only using up the exact amount of carbs that your body needs to sustain movement and none of it will get turned into stored fat. Now, the exact amount is going to differ from person to person depending on training intensity, volume, and body type. However, a general rule of thumb is that the number of carbs you should be eating should be around twice the number of grams of protein that you're consuming. If you're an endomorph who gains weight quickly, you might want to be more conservative with this approach and lower the number of carbs to maybe around 1x-1.5x your protein consumption.

Now, the conversation with carbs doesn't stop there. You also have to know that there are two different types of carbohydrates: simple and complex. The simple carbs work as fast-acting sources. They're the carbs that you need to get the job done quickly and efficiently. They're readily available and they run out just as fast. Then, there are the complex carbs. It takes longer to process the complex carbs, but they offer a more sustained steady stream of energy to the body. Think of simple carbs as energy for workouts like short sprints while complex carbs are more beneficial for marathons. Later, we'll go into detail about certain examples for both kinds of carbs.

Fat

The next item on the agenda is fat. Contrary to popular belief, eating fats don't necessarily make you fat. Again, like carbs, fat has gotten a very bad rap in the fitness community because of its name and the number of calories that it carries per gram. For one, some people think that the fat that they have around their bellies, arms, or thighs is the result of the fat that they consume from oil or meat. But that's not necessarily how fat works and that's not how your body processes fat either. Just because you eat the fatty part of a steak doesn't mean that it's going to translate into fat on your belly.

Fat is a very powerful micronutrient that helps your body absorb and process all the other essential nutrients that it needs to function properly. So, in a way, they are crucial to the muscle building process as they help your muscles absorb more protein and recover from strenuous workouts more efficiently. Fat is also responsible for improving your body's immune system and they can also be tapped as a potential energy source for whenever your body runs out of carbohydrates.

Like carbs, not all fatty food items are created equal. Fat can be categorized into two distinct types: saturated and unsaturated. Essentially, you can tell the two apart based on how they appear at room temperature. Typically, unsaturated fats take on a liquid form at room temperature while saturated fats retain their solid form. When incorporating fats into your diet, you want to make sure that you're sticking to unsaturated fats as much as possible. These are the types of fat that are responsible for providing all the positive health effects on your body's internal processes. Conversely, diets that are rich in saturated fats are often associated with diseases like stroke, cardiac disease, and hypertension.

Protein

Lastly, there is protein - every bodybuilder's favorite macro. Proteins consist of different types of amino acids. They are often referred to as the building blocks of any muscle tissue. Think of a big strong house and picture its sturdy walls and protective roof. That house wouldn't be as strong and sturdy as it is without the cement blocks that were used to fortify that structure. Protein essentially serves as the cement blocks for your body. This is why protein is immensely popular in fitness, especially for building strength and muscle.

Now, what are some of the practical benefits of protein exactly? Well, first it's about increasing strength and mass. The more protein that gets fed into your muscles, the stronger and bigger they're bound to become. This is why it's completely pointless for you to be lifting a bunch of weight at the gym but not eating the proper amount of protein to supplement it. All of your efforts will end up being wasted. Also, protein is in charge of facilitating your body's recovery process after going through vigorous workouts. It can help repair any breaks that take place in your muscle tissues and joints to make sure that you come back stronger and fitter than before you started working out. Protein is also low in calories as compared to fats. Like carbs, a single gram of protein only carries four calories. However, it's important that you still do not consume more protein than is required. If you're eating a lot of protein, but aren't doing the resistance training that necessitates a high consumption, then all of that protein will be turned into fat. You have to do strength training to create those breakages in your muscle fibers where protein can swim to and repair. If these breaks don't exist, then the protein you eat will be processed and turned into stored fat instead.

Of Calories and Metabolism

We've already touched on these two concepts in the first chapter of this book. Now, we're going to shift things up by taking a more practical and applicable approach to the ideas in this segment. Before we do that, let's go through a brief refresher. Any food that you eat carries a certain caloric value. For example, a medium-sized egg can have as much as 70 calories and a cup of rice can have around 250 calories. The reason that foods have calories is that they are made of nutrients that feed and nourish your body. The calories in your food are processed by your body and then utilized as fuel for daily function. If you eat calories in excess of any energy you're expending, then you're putting yourself in a caloric surplus. If you're not eating enough calories, then you're going into what is called a caloric deficit.

Now, how do you know how many calories you're burning in your body? That all depends on something called metabolism. This is your body's ability to take the calories you consume and convert it into energy. The higher your body's metabolism, then the more calories that you burn at any given moment. The converse is true should you have a slower level of metabolism. Given that, if you have a higher metabolism, then you would burn more daily calories than someone else with lower metabolism even though you eat the same amount of food. If you have more calories left over in your body, then you are likely to gain weight over time. If you eat fewer calories than you're using up, then you will end up losing weight.

But how do calories affect your weight gain exactly? Well, to put it to a numerical value, a single pound of fat equals around 3,500 calories. So, if over a week your total caloric deficit amounts to 3,500 calories, then you will be one pound lighter than the week prior. If you flip it and have a 3,500-calorie surplus, then you will gain a pound of fat over a week instead. When it comes to muscles, it's a little more complicated. A single pound of muscle is only composed of 700 calories. However, that doesn't mean that eating 700 calories will lead to you gaining a pound of muscle. It's estimated that you need to consume around 2700 - 3000 calories from lean protein in order to gain a pound of muscle.

Figuring Out Your Base Metabolic Rate

Now, you might be feeling a little overwhelmed right now with all of the nutrition knowledge that's been discussed so far. Don't worry. Ultimately, the only thing that you need to know about calories and metabolism is that it's a game of pluses and minuses. The more calories you have at the end of the day, the more pounds you will gain and vice-versa. Also, the higher your body's metabolism, then the more calories you will be able to burn in a day. Great. So, now that's out of the way, you need to get to work on figuring out just how many calories you're using up in a day. Sure, there are smartwatches and fitness trackers out there that may give you a rough estimate of how many calories you're using up daily. But it also pays to be able to make these computations on your own. Not everyone is going to want to shell out cash for these fitness trackers that aren't guaranteed to provide data that is 100% accurate anyway.

Before we can get to discussing the hows of computing for your base metabolic rate, we have to make sure that you understand what a base metabolic rate is and why it's important, to begin with.

The thing about your body's metabolism is that it's always at work even when you don't realize it. You might just be sitting in front of your computer or lying down in bed. Your body is still trying to convert calories into energy. Basic bodily processes like breathing, cell regeneration, blood circulation, and digestion all require energy. Most people might jump on a treadmill and see that they're burning a certain number of calories during a single running session. But the calories you burn during exercise aren't the only calories that you burn throughout the day. Your body also burns calories at other points during the day in order to sustain itself. The rate of your calorie-burn outside of exercise is referred to as your base metabolic rate.

Now, it's important for you to figure out your base metabolic rate so that you know how many calories you should be consuming in order to sustain yourself without getting fat or losing muscle. Again, if you eat too much, you might end up gaining weight. If you eat too little, your body won't recover as quickly from training sessions and you will struggle to gain lean muscle. Computing for your base metabolic rate or BMR is as simple as following this no-fuss formula:

For Women:

BMR = 655 + (9.6 × weight in kg) + (1.8 × height in cm) – (4.7 × age in years)

For Men:

BMR = 66 + (13.7 × weight [kg]) + (5 × height [cm]) – (6.8 × age [years])

What would this computation look like? Let's say you're a 29-year-old man who stands 180 cm tall and weighs 85 kg. To compute for your BMR, it's merely a matter of substituting values.

BMR = 66 + (13.7 x 85) + (5 x 180) - (6.8 x 29)

   = 66+ (1164.5) + (900) - (197.2)

   = 1,933.3

So, based on these computations in this example, you would be burning 1,933 calories daily outside of any additional calories burned from exercise. Again, BMR doesn't take into consideration any amount of training that you might be doing. If you really want to dial in on how many calories you're burning daily, then you have to first assess how active you are. Try to fit yourself into one of the following categories:

Sedentary - minimal to no exercise (multiply BMR by 1.2)

Lightly active - light exercise 1-3 times a week (multiply BMR by 1.375)

Moderately active - moderate exercise 3-5 times a week (multiply BMR by 1.55)

Very active - hard exercise 6-7 times a week (multiply BMR by 1.725)

Extra active - very hard exercise 6-7 times a week (or if your profession is physical in nature like construction work, athlete, etc.) (multiply BMR by 1.9)

Of course, these are just rough estimates. It's not an exact science. The numbers might be skewed depending on a variety of factors. Take whatever results you get from these computations as ballpark figures that you should be aiming for and adjust your training/diet plan accordingly. If you see that the results are good, then stick with it. If you feel like your computations are off, then make the necessary adjustments.

Caloric Surplus or Deficit?

You might already have a fairly good understanding of how many calories you're burning each day based on your body type, age, gender, and level of physical activity. You were able to compute your base metabolic rate and you also multiplied that amount based on how much physical activity you engage in over a week. Now, it's time for you to try to figure out how much you should be feeding yourself. Depending on your relationship with food, you may or may not like what you're about to read here. For some people, eating large amounts of food (especially bland healthy food like greens and chicken breast) can be a struggle. For many, cutting out bad food like sweets and junk food can be an even bigger tragedy. However, no one ever said that getting the body of your dreams was going to be easy.

In this segment, we are going to delve deeper into the idea of caloric surpluses and caloric deficits. What are the benefits of either and when are they useful? Ultimately, it's as simple as determining what your goals are. If you are an ectomorph or a mesomorph with a relatively skinny frame, then you should look into having a caloric surplus. Your body is burning so much fuel and energy to compensate for your level of physical activity. If you want to build lean muscle, then it's important that you feed your body adequately with healthy lean proteins and complex carbs. You don't want to be going into a caloric deficit because this will hinder the process of hypertrophy in your body. However, your approaches to caloric surpluses should be different. If you're an ectomorph, you have a little more wiggle room and a higher margin for error with regard to how many excess calories you can consume daily without getting fat. If you're a mesomorph, you want to be very careful to not overdo it with your caloric surplus. A general rule of thumb is to not exceed an excess of 500 calories per day so that you maximize muscle growth and minimize fat gain.

If you're an endomorph, then your margin for error is a lot slimmer as compared to a mesomorph and ectomorph with regard to staving off fat. It's so easy for you to gain weight even when you're training really hard at the gym. While it's okay in some instances for you to go into a caloric surplus, it's not an absolute necessity. Sometimes, you would be better off at just balancing out your calories burned and calories consumed entirely. In some cases, endomorphs can still even gain muscle while going into a caloric deficit so long as they are getting most of their calories from protein. However, if you really want to go into a caloric surplus, make sure that you don't exceed 300 excess calories daily and incorporate more cardio into your training.

Structuring Your Diet Plan around the Three Macros

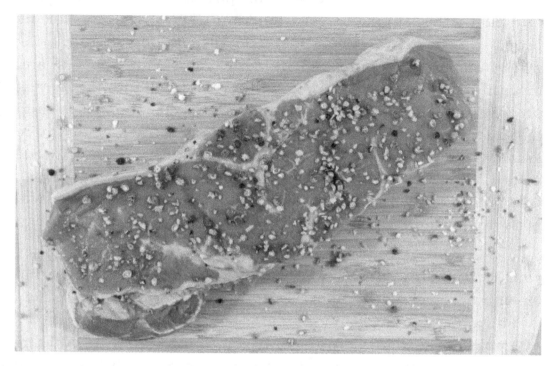

You might be growing a little frustrated over how theoretical a lot of these concepts have been so far. You already know about calories burned and calories consumed. You're already familiar with surpluses and deficits. But how is that knowledge going to translate to the amount of food that you should be eating? In order for you to create an effective diet plan for yourself, then you need to utilize your knowledge of the three macronutrients.

What Should Your Plate Look Like?

It would be ideal if you pay close attention to every single nutrient that goes into your body. However, it's also quite impractical. You don't always have to stay on top of how much sodium, potassium, or vitamin C that you're getting with every meal. The more practical way of paying attention to your nutrition is by looking at your macronutrients. There are some people who want to take a more detailed approach to dieting where they really count the numeric values for calories and macronutrients. This is a great way to really drill into the dieting process, but it isn't necessary. Sure, there are a lot of fitness and dieting apps along the way that can help you track what you're eating and how much of it translates to certain nutritional values. However, all that really matters is that you eat enough that makes you feel like you can sustain your physical performance and functionality every day.

If you want to take a more hands-on approach to tracking your food, then go ahead. Make use of a traditional food journal or embrace technology and use apps like MyFitnessPal to help you document your food more intensively. But for a lot of people, a simple eye test would suffice. If you're interested in building lean muscle while staving off fat, try to maintain a 40-30-30 ratio for calories that you consume in a day. What this means is that of the total amount of calories that you eat daily, 40% should be made up of protein sources, while 30% should come from each of the other two macros, fats, and carbs. To illustrate this further in numbers, imagine that you have a prescribed diet plan of 2500 daily calories in order for you to have a healthy caloric surplus.

40% of 2500 = 1000 calories

30% of 2500 = 750 calories

Given that, you should aim for a macro distribution of 1000 calories worth of protein, 750 calories worth of fats, and another 750 calories from carbs.

However, these values are not absolute. Again, there are plenty of variables that come into play here. Mostly, the ideal distribution of macros here all depends on your goals. If you're looking to trim down, it might be best for you to opt for a higher protein count. So, maybe you can go for a 50-25-25 or 50-30-20 breakdown. It all depends on how your body will respond to certain dietary formats. You have the freedom and wiggle room to play around here to see what works for you.

Keep in mind that as you progress in your bodybuilding journey, your body is going to respond to food intake differently over time. A lot of the time, you will find that you will hit certain plateaus in your fitness journey. If this is the case, the first thing that you have to do is adjust your training. Take note of the principle of progressive overload. You need to be making your workouts more and more challenging as you get stronger. If that still doesn't work, then you might have to tweak your diet. If you're not progressing as quickly as before with regards to building muscle, then you might have to up your calorie or protein intake. Perhaps you're getting a little pudgy and gaining a little bit of unwanted fat. This might be a sign for you to lower your calorie intake and carbohydrate consumption.

Best Food for Carbohydrates

Ideally, carbs should cover around 30% of your total caloric intake every day. However, not all carbs are created equal. You want to make sure that you are sourcing your carbs from whole foods that add more nutritional value to your diet plan.

300 calories from steel-cut oats are not the same as 300 calories from ice cream. One contains a lot of healthy fiber that will help your digestive system while the other is loaded with unnecessary sugar that will give you insulin spikes. Whole foods tend to also make you feel fuller for longer. This means that you won't have those random cravings in the middle of the day for unhealthy junk. Here are a few examples of the best food sources for carbohydrates:

- steel-cut oats
- whole wheat bread
- brown or red rice
- whole wheat pasta
- green leafy vegetables (lettuce, cabbage, spinach, kale, etc.)
- tomatoes
- bell peppers
- quinoa
- sweet potatoes

Best Food for Fat

For the most part, you just want to stay away from food items that have a high amount of trans fats in them. They are referred to as bad fats because they are notorious for negatively impacting a person's cardiac health and overall immune system. Instead, shoot for generous amounts of unsaturated fats and moderate amounts of saturated fats. These are fats that carry a lot of antioxidants and natural nutrients that will help regulate your body's internal processes.

Unsaturated Fats

- olive oil

- nuts
- nut butters
- peanuts
- seeds (pumpkin, sesame, etc.)
- fatty fish (salmon, mackerel, etc.)
- vegetable oils (canola, corn, sunflower, etc.)-avocadoes

Saturated Fats

- cheese
- butter
- cream
- fat from meat
- coconut oil
- palm oil

Best Food for Protein

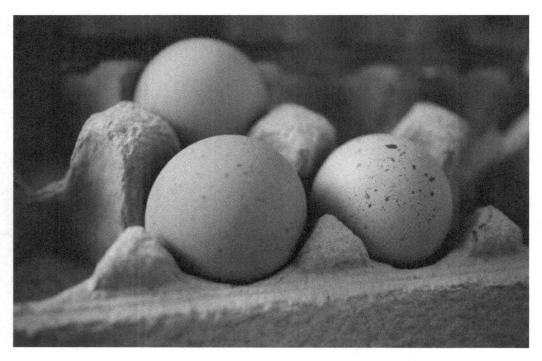

Lastly, of course, there is protein. You already know that protein serves as the cement blocks that will build the foundation of your body's musculature. So, in any type of bodybuilding-focused diet, you want to make sure that you are getting a generous dose of healthy lean protein from natural food sources. Most of the time, you can get protein from meats like beef, chicken, pork, and fish. However, it's also possible to get protein if you're on a plant-based diet. Here are some of the most common sources of protein from food:

- Eggs
- milk
- cheese
- chicken

- pork
- turkey
- beef
- fish
- nuts
- beans
- legumes
- yogurt, etc.

Top Foods to AVOID at All Costs

Discipline is a very important trait to master when you're trying to build your optimal physique. A lot of people tend to get hung up on the aspect of discipline that focuses on establishing new routines and adopting new habits. However, not a lot of people realize that discipline also has to do with getting rid of bad habits that might be detrimental to you pursuing your goals. There might be certain food items in your current diet plan that you need to eliminate altogether if you really want to maximize your strength and resistance training endeavors. Here are some common culprits of food items that might keep you from achieving your goals:

Alcoholic Beverages

As painful as it might be, you're going to have to part ways with your favorite beers, whiskeys, tequilas, and vodka cocktails for a while. The sad truth is that alcoholic beverages can inhibit your body's ability to process the nutrients that it needs to sustain itself. This means that the muscles that you break from resistance training aren't going to be repaired as efficiently with protein when you have alcohol running through your bloodstream.

On top of that, you are taking on a lot of unnecessary calories when you go out on a night of binge drinking with friends. A single serving of beer can often contain as much as 150 or even 200 calories. You might opt for harder liquors that have relatively lower calorie counts, but if you mix them in with other ingredients like sweeteners or sodas, then it's all moot. An occasional beer every now and then isn't going to be so bad for your body. Just try to make sure that you limit the alcohol intake as much as possible. If you can, try eliminating it from your diet altogether.

Refined or Added Sugars

In general, food that is high in refined or added sugars add very little value to your body's nutritional intake. Of course, it can be very tempting to reward yourself with a delicious donut or a pint of ice cream after a hard workout. However, you would also be effectively undoing a lot of the progress that you make in the gym. Instead of getting leaner and gaining more muscle, you are only adding sugars to your body which will get converted into stored body fat and cause you to crash and burn. Instead of rewarding yourself with sweet treats after a workout, opt for healthier options like a fruit smoothie or some low-carb protein bars.

At the end of the day, there's no denying that a good old chocolate bar is going to taste much better than a bowl of kale. But no one ever said that dieting was going to be easy. Try to limit your consumption of food items like sodas, sugary sports drinks, sugary coffee beverages, ice cream, cake, donuts, cookies, potato chips, and the like. They're okay for occasional treats, but you shouldn't be making it a habit of consuming these items consistently.

Deep-Fried Food Items

Just because chicken is filled with a lot of protein doesn't mean that you should be eating buckets of fried chicken for every meal. Working hard at the gym doesn't give you an excuse to line up at KFC every day. The truth is that these deep-fried food items like fried chicken and french fries are laden with a lot of unnecessary calories that come from fat sources like oil and carb sources like breading and flour. On top of that, these deep-fried items can promote inflammation in your body and can slow down the muscle recovery process.

Common examples of deep-fried food items are fish fingers, chicken nuggets, fried chicken, potato chips, french fries, onion rings, corn dogs, and more.

Best Supplements for Bodybuilders

Now, it's time to discuss the idea of supplementation. The first thing that you have to know about supplementation is that it isn't necessarily a requirement in order for you to build lean muscle. If you really commit to having a clean and healthy diet, then you are going to find success in your goals in fitness. However, for a lot of people, one can only get so far on food alone. There are just some people who will find it difficult to stuff themselves with pounds of lean chicken breast every day in order to meet protein requirements. This is exactly where supplementation comes in.

There are a lot of people who might be hesitant to try supplementation at first because of a certain reputation that these substances might carry. There are many novices who might lump healthy and natural supplements along with performance-enhancing drugs like steroids. These are not the same. It's important to emphasize that it's perfectly safe to make use of health supplements in proper moderation. Your relationship with supplements should be the same one that you have with your food. You should only be taking in what your body needs to perform optimally. Also, supplements should be seen as something that accompanies a proper diet based on food. They shouldn't be acting as meal replacements. As much as possible, you want to source your nutrients from whole foods that are as natural as can be.

Having said that, you can still benefit from cycling supplements into your daily dietary rotation. You just have to know what specific supplements to look out for, how much of them you need, and what purposes they might serve in your training regimen. In terms of bodybuilding, here are some of the top supplements that you might want to invest in.

Whey Protein

The first supplement that you want to invest in is whey protein. This is essentially one of the most popular supplements out there for bodybuilders. This is because of the fundamental bodybuilding aspects that protein has on the body. Ideally, whey protein is a product that is consumed immediately after a hard workout. Preferably, within 30 minutes. This is because whey is a fast-acting protein and is absorbed by the muscles quickly. A lot of modern whey protein manufacturers also market products in a variety of flavors. Whey protein usually comes in a powder form and can be mixed in with other ingredients like milk, juices, or blended fruits. This can make whey protein a perfect go-to treat or reward after a difficult workout.

Casein Protein

Casein protein is another kind of protein supplement that usually comes in a powder form as well. However, it differs from whey protein in terms of the time that it takes to be processed. Whey protein needs to be absorbed into the body within 30 minutes after a hard workout in order for one to yield optimal benefits. This is because whey mostly acts within a short amount of time. With casein, it's different. It's a much slower process. Most people drink casein protein before going to sleep. This is so that your body is receiving a constant flow of protein all throughout the night. Studies have also shown that the muscle recovery process heightens during the sleep stage.

Weight Gainers

If you are someone who gains weight easily like an endomorph or a mesomorph, then you might not want to invest in this product. However, if you are an ectomorph who struggles to pack on the calories that are required to build muscle, then you can try out weight gainers. Usually, these are powdered substances that are loaded up with a lot of protein, either whey or casein. However, aside from that, they are also loaded with carbohydrates to add to the calories per serving. Again, make sure that this supplement is only used alongside a healthy diet plan that revolves around real food. It shouldn't serve as a meal replacement.

BCAA (Branched Chain Amino Acids)

Typically, branched-chain amino acids or BCAA consist of three essential acids that are crucial for building muscle: leucine, isoleucine, and valine. Typically, you would be able to source these acids in incremental amounts through meats, poultry, dairy, and fish. This is essentially a supplement that is meant for people who don't eat enough protein from whole foods in their diet. Again, not everyone is going to be happy with stuffing themselves with chunks of chicken breast or tuna for every meal. This is where supplements like BCAA come in to help you get the nutrients that you need without having to eat an uncomfortable amount of food.

Creatine

Aside from whey protein, there are plenty of bodybuilders who will say that creatine is their go-to supplement. First of all, creatine is responsible for taking all of the water that you drink and feeding it into your muscles. Almost 80% of your muscles are made up of water and creatine helps make sure that your muscles always stay hydrated. Aside from that, it is also responsible for providing energy to your muscles so that they are always optimized for peak physical performance whenever you're working out. It's a lot easier to build strength and mass through a regular intake of creatine. However, there are detractors who will say that creatine can damage your kidneys or liver because it takes all of the water you drink away from these organs and feeds it into your muscles instead. This is why it's important that you stay hydrated and drink a lot of water whenever you are on a creatine cycle.

Omega-3 Fatty Acids

You might be familiar with Omega-3 Fatty Acids as those nutrients that are always found in fish oil gels. This is a supplement that is particularly popular among the elderly as it is often marketed as a product that helps with joint pains and aches. However, more than just strengthening your joints, fish oil can also help the recovery process by decreasing the inflammation in your muscles. This means that you will tend to feel less sore after a hard workout and it will be easier for you to exert more effort in the gym the next day.

Caffeine

Yes, caffeine. Not a lot of people may realize that caffeine is a very popular dietary supplement for athletes and people who stay active in general. Caffeine is especially popular among bodybuilders for two reasons. One, it increases the body's metabolism. This means that it helps the body burn more fat while at rest. The other reason that caffeine is so popular is that it provides athletes with the energy and stamina that they need to sustain difficult workouts. Marathoners and endurance athletes are popularly known to take caffeine prior to a race. However, bodybuilders also usually take caffeine prior to a heavy lifting session in order to provide more energy to the muscles.

The Best Nutrition Secrets, Tips, and Tricks

Nutrition is a complicated topic. It's possible that you're feeling a little overwhelmed with everything that has been discussed so far, and that's okay. This is not something you should expect to master in a day. These are all very complex ideas that you need to gradually integrate into your daily life. It's not something that you can just fully absorb in one go and then be done with. Given that, perhaps it's best to summarize all of the knowledge into bite-sized tips and tricks that you can apply to your everyday life.

Again, your success is ultimately going to be determined by the habits that you practice every day. If you just try to apply these simple secrets and tips to your life on a consistent basis, you are bound to see results. And you won't even have to wait too long to feel like you're progressing.

Prioritize Real Food

Again, it's important that you prioritize real food. And when we say real food, we mean food that undergoes the least amount of processing as possible. Avoid overly processed goods such as canned meats, bagged chips, chocolate bars, and the like. These are not real food and they aren't going to help you get the body that you want. As much as possible, try to focus on sourcing your meals from meats and plants. Try to keep it as clean as possible.

Don't Be Afraid of Supplements

Now that you know that you have to prioritize real food always, let's talk about the value of supplements. Ultimately, you want to prioritize real food as much as you can. However, there will be times where you just can't get the nutrients that you need from whole foods alone. This is where supplementation can really help you out. For instance, you might be reaching your caloric limit for the day, but you still need some extra protein. A nice glass of whey protein can help you meet your protein needs without you having to find a chicken to munch on at the end of the day or after a workout.

Drink Lots of Water

Again, water is life. Literally. You have to make sure that you stay hydrated whenever you're looking to build muscle. For one, your muscles are made out of water. In fact, your entire body is made out of water. You want to make sure that your body is hydrated so that it would be able to function properly. Also, staying hydrated helps your cells regenerate faster and it can aid in muscle recovery as well. It can also be very dangerous to your kidneys if you are consuming a lot of protein without drinking an ample amount of water. Eating too much protein and not enough water can compromise the integrity of your kidneys.

Track Your Food Intake

You definitely want to keep track of the food that you're eating. There is no way that you would be able to maximize your potential and achieve the goals that you want just by winging it. Sure, there are some people who are experienced enough to know how much they should be eating without keeping a food journal. However, this only comes through consistent practice and experience. If you're a novice and you're just starting out, you really need to take the time to track what you're eating as accurately as possible. This might seem like it's a lot of work to do, but no one ever said that this was going to be easy.

Plan Your Meals

Tracking your meals might seem like such a hassle. However, if you engage in meal planning and preparation, then everything becomes a lot easier and simpler. All it takes is just one day of a week for you to sit down and write all the meals that you'll be eating over the course of seven days. Write everything down and include all the major meals along with your snacks. This is beneficial for numerous reasons. For one, it makes the grocery shopping process a lot simpler. You will only end up buying the ingredients that you need for your meal plan. Next, it will be easier for you to track your meals and caloric intake when you've planned them out beforehand. It's also going to help keep you from overeating or undereating throughout the week whenever you have a plan to follow.

Make Adjustments Whenever Necessary

The diet plan that you start with isn't necessarily going to be the diet plan that you stick with for the rest of your life. You have to understand that your body is going to go through some significant changes as you get older and fitter. This is why it isn't always going to respond to a particular diet plan the same way forever. It's important that you continually reassess the effectiveness of your diet plan. If you notice that you aren't getting the proper results, then be open to tweaking your diet a little bit to accommodate for the changes in your body or workout routine.

When Unsure, Eat Meat and Vegetables

There will be times where you won't be able to figure out what you should be eating. This is especially true whenever you find yourself having nights out with friends or family at restaurants. You might be forced to stray away from your meal plan and order something on the spot. Don't worry. Just remember that you can never go wrong with lean meats and vegetables. When in doubt, order a salad and a meat of some kind. Make sure that there is a minimal amount of sauce and dressing. This way, you know you are still eating clean even when you're eating outside.

Fibrous Carbs Over Sugar

Carbs are not the enemy here. Hopefully, you will have learned that when you were reading about the macros and the different roles that they play in building muscle and staying healthy. You should always look to incorporate carbs into your diet to a certain extent. However, whenever you do eat carbs, always try to prioritize fibrous carbs over sugary ones. Go for carbs like wheat and grains because they help aid in your digestion and body's processing of nutrients. Sugar is just going to give you unsustainable energy and unwanted body fat.

Avoid Alcohol

Just avoid alcohol. Avoid drinking beers and wines because they're loaded with a lot of calories and carbohydrates. Also, avoid drinking cocktails because they usually have a lot of unwanted carbs and sugars in them as well. Hard liquors might seem okay because they are low in calories, but they can really compromise your body's ability to absorb protein. So, just try to avoid alcohol to the best of your abilities. Of course, this doesn't mean that you can't have alcohol for as long as you live. Which brings us to our next and final tip...

Treat Yourself (Sometimes)

Have an occasional cheat day. Go ahead. Life isn't worth living if you're not having fun. At the end of the day, you really need to learn to enjoy the process if you're going to find success in it. There's nothing enjoyable about being strict and always disciplining yourself. Sure, you're going to find a lot of success that way. However, you should never pursue success at the cost of your own happiness. This is why it's good if you have an occasional cheat day. Even as a reward system, this can be a very good practice to have in your fitness journey. For example, you can reward yourself with a scoop of ice cream after a week's worth of strict dieting. Maybe you can go out on a one-night drinking binge after gaining 5 lbs. of muscle to celebrate. Just make sure that these treats are done very rarely. They might not be good for your body, but they're good for your soul.

Final Thoughts

By now, you should be convinced that diets are very important in determining how your body is going to respond to training stimuli. You are never going to progress as quickly or as efficiently as you should be in the gym if you're not supplementing your workouts with proper nutrition habits. As tempting as it might be to just indulge in a diet of pasta, pizza, burgers, donuts, cookies, ice cream, and beer all of the time, you're going to have to develop your sense of discipline. To reiterate a point that was made at the start of this chapter, you can't outrun a bad diet. If you're continually eating junk, then your body is never going to achieve everything that it's designed to achieve.

It can be so easy to fall into the trap of thinking that just because you're working hard at the gym, this means that you can eat whatever you want. This is absolutely the wrong mindset to have when it comes to designing your diet plan. True fitness is a healthy collaboration of both physical training and nutrition. You need to marry these to concepts in order for you to achieve optimal health and wellness. A failure to conflate a good training regimen with proper diets can result in suboptimal results. It's just that simple.

Hopefully, this chapter will have given you good insight and sufficient motivation to pursue a healthier lifestyle in the realms of the kitchen. Not all battles take place on the race track or in the boxing ring. Master the art of proper dieting and nutrition to win the ultimate war against unwanted body fat.

Chapter 4

Rest and Recovery

It's not always just about working hard. Fitness and nutrition aren't only about the work you put in the gym or your dieting discipline. It's also about how you take care of your body in terms of rest and recovery. Sure, it can get pretty addicting to just spend all day every day at the gym when you're just starting out. This is especially true if you've managed to find a lot of success instantly. That success can become addicting to the point where you crave it over and over again like a drug. So, since you've found success by working hard at the gym, you think that you can get more of it by spending time at the gym. In theory, this can be true. However, in all practicality, you're only human and you need to rest. In fact, you might be doing more harm than good to your body if you don't give it the proper care that it needs in order for you to carry on towards achieving your fitness goals.

This chapter is going to turn the spotlight towards the importance of recovery, sleep, and just taking care of your body in general. Whenever you start working out, it can be pretty amazing to witness all of the remarkable things your body can do. You would never be able to imagine yourself lifting certain weights or defining particular muscle groups until you see them happening. There are some people who go their whole lives thinking that they could never deadlift twice their bodyweight. And it's only because they never think to even try it. So, when you see that your body is performing these amazing feats, it can be tempting to just keep on pushing. However, the problem with that is that you end up putting yourself in danger of injury whenever you don't allow yourself the chance to rest or recover.

There are many ways to approach keeping your body safe and primed for action in the gym every day. A lot of it has to do with certain exercises or habits that you can employ, such as mandatory rest days and

supplementation. Sleep is also an important factor that you need to take into consideration here. Try working out while running on less than four hours of sleep and compare it to when you work out after feeling fully rested. You will inevitably find a significant difference in how you feel.

Aside from allowing yourself a chance to recover, there is also the matter of making sure that you keep yourself safe from injuries through prehab. Remember that in medicine, prevention is always better than the cure. Don't wait for yourself to get injured or become overworked before you start doing soft tissue work or stretching. These are all concepts that are going to be discussed in greater detail all throughout this chapter. Again, it's not just about going hard at the gym and being disciplined in the kitchen all the time. This is the other less exciting, less glamorous, and more boring aspect of fitness. However, there is no denying just how important these lessons are.

The Importance of Rest and Recovery

All of the successful people you will ever meet in your life will tell you that their success is built by hard work. No exceptions. You can never achieve your grandest goals and dreams unless you put forth the willingness to work hard and suffer for them. It can be so easy to get lost in the romanticism of pouring your blood, sweat, and tears into achieving what you want. This is a concept that is often sensationalized in contemporary media. But do you know the part that rarely gets advertised? Rest and recovery. Picture a superhero movie. You are always so used to seeing Captain America and the Avengers in action fighting against the evilest villains in the world. You see them fight and claw their way to victory. It's very exciting. But what don't you see? You never see Captain America taking a nap. You don't see Batman taking the time to do mobility work for his muscles. You will never see Superman say that he needs a rest day.

Wake up. You're not a superhero and you don't live in fantasy land. You might feel like your body is capable of a lot, and that's a good thing. It always pays to be confident. However, you have to make sure that you don't overstretch yourself here. You are capable of great things, that's true. However, you also need to rest and recover from greatness every once in a while.

When you go to the gym, you are expected to give it your best every single time. And as you engage in hard training, your muscles will break themselves down further and further. You've already learned about this in previous chapters. You know that breaking your muscles down is an important step in the process of hypertrophy. As you break your muscles down, you inevitably become weaker in the short-term only to come out stronger in the long-term. However, getting long-term muscle gains is not achieved merely through hard work at the gym or through proper dieting. There is another dimension to that: rest.

Again, you get weaker in the short-term after a tough training session. Rest and recovery are responsible for making sure that you come out stronger than ever before. When you take the time to rest, you are giving your muscles a chance to heal from being broken down and beaten up. Once you recover through resting, your muscles will feel refreshed and equipped to move heavier loads at more rapid paces. You also already know that hard training can lead to a number of physiological benefits for the human body. Improved blood flow, heart health, respiratory function, digestion, and others are among the benefits you stand to gain from exercising regularly. However, if you don't allow an ample recovery period for your body in between training sessions, these benefits become compromised. Besides that, engaging in what is referred to as overtraining can lead to experiencing performance plateaus and injuries.

What is Overtraining?

One general principle that you can apply to any aspect of life is that anything done in excess is bad - even things that you might think are good for you. This, of course, includes training and exercise. Now, it can be very difficult to define what overtraining is because it's a sensation that can vary from person to person. A professional runner might be capable of covering 100 miles per week, while the average joe would only be capable of 20 within the same span. Anything beyond that would be overtraining for Joe and just another regular work week for the professional. It's all relative. In this segment of the book, you will be given insights into how you can personally assess whether you are overtraining or not.

There are many factors that can influence a person's capacity for training. Of course, a lot of it has to do with that person's training experience or current level of physical fitness. However, there are also more nuanced factors such as genetics, age, muscle composition, diet, and whatnot. A general rule of thumb is that an average of around 48 to 72 hours of recovery is required in between intense strength training sessions. However, this length of recovery can lessen for those who can gradually increase their workload capacity.

Signs of Overtraining

Now, how would you be able to tell if you are overtraining? It would be nice if you got yourself a licensed professional to oversee your training so that you wouldn't have to worry about details like these. However, if you don't have the luxury of getting personalized instruction from a professional, then you might need to do these assessments on your own. Fortunately for you, it's not that complicated of a process. At the end of the day, the best person to determine whether your body is overly stressed or not is yourself. There are a few signs or symptoms of overtraining that you can be on the lookout for whenever you feel like you're overdoing it at the gym. These signs can be divided into physical and emotional/behavioral classifications.

Physical

- persistent muscle soreness
- joint pain
- fever
- Elevated blood pressure
- elevated heart rate
- decreased appetite
- unintended weight loss

Emotional/Behavioral

- irritability
- insomnia
- depression
- anxiety
- elevated heart rate
- lack of motivation

The Importance of Sleep

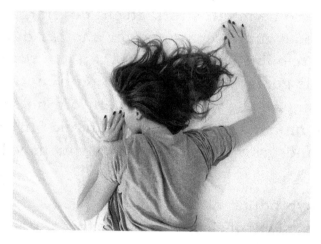

Many working adults will know that sleep is a very precious resource that not many people will have the luxury of getting enough of. Too many times, people will take not just the quantity of their sleep, but also the quality of their sleep for granted in favor of productivity throughout the day. However, while it might make more sense to stay up a couple of extra hours at night to get more things done, it can actually be counterintuitive to your desires to be more productive. In fact, compelling evidence suggests that going multiple days in a row without getting adequate sleep can lead to you feeling groggy and fatigued throughout the day. Therefore, it will be much harder for you to stay focused and motivated to accomplish specific tasks.

It's the same with bodybuilding as well. You might not think much of the amount of time that you devote to sleep. However, you may not realize that the quantity (and quality) of your sleep can have a significant impact on two things: the way that your muscles repair, recover, and grow along with the way that you perform while you're training. Essentially, the time you sleep is when your body goes into a deep hibernation and self repair mode. Your mind shuts itself down and focuses on repairing the body and preparing it for another day of the usual activities. You're doing so much more than just resting your eyes and brain while going to sleep. You are rejuvenating your entire body. If you compromise your sleep, then your muscles won't end up getting as much recovery as they should. In the end, they won't repair and grow as efficiently as you may have initially wished.

As a byproduct of not allowing your body to recover properly due to a lack of sleep, you can expect suboptimal output and performance whenever you put your body to work. Your muscles never got the chance to repair and rejuvenate themselves properly. So, you might end up still feeling sore and tired when you go to the gym. As a result, you wouldn't be able to maximize your workout because of how fatigued you feel. It's important that you really understand why sleep is important and how you should be integrating proper sleeping habits into your routine.

Understanding the Sleep Cycles

It's been mentioned a couple of times that it's not just the quantity of sleep that you need to be paying attention to. It's just as important that you take note of the quality of your sleep. And before you can really understand what that means, you have to learn about the various sleep cycles.

When you go to sleep at night, there are various stages that you go through. It's a cycle; a repetitive process that has you going from being awake to being immersed in a truly deep sleep over and over again until you wake up. Most people can go through three to five cycles of sleep per night, but it varies from person to person.

Stage 1: Awake

This is usually the stage where you're still slightly awake but you're gradually drifting off to sleep. You might have experienced this when you catch yourself dozing off in the middle of watching TV or while reading a book. During this stage, your senses start to lull themselves and your heart rate begins to slow down.

You're not entirely asleep, but you're not fully awake either. This is the transitory period of you shifting from a conscious state to an unconscious one.

Stage 2: Light Sleep

The second stage of sleep sees your brain and muscles winding themselves down. Your brain activity decreases significantly and your muscles will relax to the point where they lie in a completely static state. Usually, you enter the light sleep stage around 15 to 30 minutes after falling asleep. This is the stage of sleep where you are most easily awakened either by outside noise or physical prompts. Hence, it's called the light sleep stage.

Stage 3: Deep Sleep

The deep sleep stage is the one you want to get the most out of when you talk about bodybuilding and muscle recovery. Deep sleep is the quality sleep that you always want to aim for when it comes to repairing your body. This is the stage of sleep where your brain and muscle activity really goes down to the point where the activity is practically nonexistent. Your heart rate is also probably at its lowest possible point during this time. Usually, people enter a deep sleep stage within 45 minutes to an hour of falling asleep. If you get woken up from a deep sleep, you will feel very groggy and disoriented. You wouldn't automatically be able to discern your environment and it will take a while for your mind to orient itself with what's going on.

Stage 4: REM or Rapid Eye Movement

Try observing your pets whenever they go to sleep, especially your dogs. You might see that they're moving their eyes around rapidly even though they're closed. This is a sign that they've fallen into the REM stage of sleep. This is typically the age of sleep where your brain starts becoming active again and triggers your eyes to move around involuntarily. This is also the stage of sleep when your dreams take place. Most people's nightly sleeping time is around 25% of REM sleep. During this stage, your muscles will become paralyzed and your heart rate will gradually rise.

Negative Effects of Sleep Deprivation

Sleep deprivation is one thing that you always want to avoid when you're trying to live a healthier and fitter lifestyle. Whenever you don't get enough sleep at night, you will feel the negative effects almost instantly the moment you wake up. Depriving yourself of sleep every once in a while is one thing. However, if you do it consistently, then you're going to feel the significant weight of these negative effects more immensely. It's not just about feeling sleepy or tired all throughout the day. There are other physical, mental, and emotional effects that take place whenever you lack sleep as well.

As a bodybuilder, you already know that lacking sleep can slow down the muscle building and recovery process. On top of that, it can also lead to poorer neurological fitness. This means that neurological aspects of fitness like balance, accuracy, timing, and coordination are likely to be compromised whenever you lack sleep. In addition, sleep deprivation also promotes inflammation in the body. This means that swollen muscles will stay swollen for longer and will make you feel more sore than necessary.

Other negative effects that are associated with sleep deprivation include unintended weight fluctuations, mood swings, sugar cravings, lack of focus, and a weaker immune system. Working out while being deprived of sleep can also leave you being more prone to injuries.

The Importance of "Pre"hab

This entire chapter has been dedicated to principles that are focused on taking care of your body as you continually put it through various stress-inducing environments and conditions. That's exactly how you should see working out and dieting. They are stressful conditions that you put your body through in order to harden it and induce self-development. However, it's not good to just always be exposing yourself to such stressful conditions without taking the time to just take care of yourself as well. Remember that the goal here is to participate in the whole marathon. It's not an all-out sprint right out of the gate. You need to make sure that you are playing the long game.

Your days don't always have to be spent lifting heavy weights. You want to work hard, but you shouldn't be working yourself to muscle failure every single time.

This would be the quickest way to get yourself to a physical therapist's clinic for treatment. When building the body of your dreams, the last thing that you would want is to get sidelined for a prolonged period because of an injury. It's not just about safely executing the movements at the gym. It has more to do with what you're doing outside of your regular working sets.

This segment of the chapter is going to delve deeper into the idea of mobility and active recovery days. Just because you want to build muscle doesn't mean your exercise routine should be totally composed of resistance training exercises. Yes, recovery through sleep is important, but that's not the only thing that you can do to make sure that your body is always primed and ready for a hard workout.

Understanding Mobility as a Tool for Injury Prevention

You probably aren't going to get as many likes on Instagram if you post a video of yourself foam rolling instead of you lifting heavy weights. Mobility will never be as flashy or as exciting as actual strength and resistance training, but that shouldn't take away from its importance. Mobility is a very important aspect of fitness that you should incorporate into your routine even though it's not something that everyone likes to talk about. Now, what is mobility exactly? A lot of people seem to confuse mobility with flexibility even when the two are different. Flexibility is the ability of your muscle to stretch or elongate to a certain length. On the other hand, mobility is your body's ability to maintain strength and control while expanding your range of motion. Anyone who is flexible enough can touch their toes without bending their knees. But a person who is mobile would be able to get into a deep squat without having their muscles collapse or give in.

Now, why is mobility important for you as a bodybuilder? It all has to do with you maintaining strength and control as you engage in various explosive movements that are involved with resistance training. There are some people who might be able to bench press their bodyweight. But if you ask these same people to squat with their hip creases getting below the knee, they will cry out in pain. This might prevent that person from getting the potential strength gains that one might earn from engaging in the full range of motion for a movement. If you're doing just a half squat because your lack of mobility prevents you from going the full range of motion, then you are effectively limiting the potency of the movement. You aren't engaging as many muscle groups as you should and your strength gains will be impacted. So, that's one aspect of how mobility can be beneficial for you as a bodybuilder.

Another reason why mobility is important is that it will save you from potential injuries. Too often, athletes who lack proper mobility and who push themselves in training will end up getting tears in their muscles or ligaments. This is because they push their bodies beyond their capacity and the stimuli become too much for the body to handle. There's a reason why immobile people feel pain whenever they are made to squat or fully extend a press overhead. There's something wrong that's going on with their joints and fascia that is preventing them from doing the movement pain-free. Whether as a result of adrenaline or sheer will, some athletes would be able to push past that pain and execute these movements despite their lack of mobility. That pain is supposed to serve as a safeguard or a limiter. But once an athlete continuously pushes past that pain, the body just gives up.

There are various ways in which you might choose to go about improving your mobility. One common method of building mobility is doing light range-of motion exercises or dynamic stretches. These are different from static stretches where someone holds a stretch for a prolonged period of time. These range-of motion exercises or dynamic stretches are more kinetic in nature and they require constant movement. They are designed to activate muscles and loosen up tight spots, especially those that are found near joints. Another way of improving mobility is by doing soft tissue work whether through foam rolling or by using a lacrosse ball. Think of your muscles as something that is made up of tiny little threads called muscle fibers. Whenever you do resistance training, these threads become stressed and they can sometimes get entangled. These entangled threads can lead to you experiencing discomfort or having a limited range of motion when you exercise. You can make use of tools like foam rollers, massage guns, or lacrosse balls to help loosen and untangle these muscle fibers so that you regain full range of motion again. You may also use the services of a licensed massage therapist who can work on these problem areas on your body for you.

Active Recovery Days

Being a bodybuilder doesn't mean that you should just be doing bodybuilding exercises every day. Your body needs a break from that particular stimulus in order for it to recover and come back stronger. There are even some people who stick to a training regimen for too long to the point that their bodies acclimate to that routine. When that happens, they experience a plateau in their progress because their bodies aren't responding to the training stimuli in the same manner as before. This is why it's important for you to break your routine up by incorporating occasional rest days or cross training. If you feel like you have too much energy to go a full day without doing any kind of exercise, then you can have an active recovery day.

Of course, the first option would be for you to just have an all-out rest day. Take one day away from the gym and don't do any exercise at all. During rest days, it's important that you still stay strict on your diet, especially when you're trying to lose fat by going into a caloric deficit. Remember that you're not burning as many calories during these days because you're not going to the gym.

Another option that you can take is by doing an active recovery day. This means that you take the time to do some form of exercise that is less intense and has a different stimulus as your regular routine. This could be anything from shooting hoops in your backyard or doing a quick yoga session. You can even just take some time to do some foam rolling and myofascial release on yourself to work on your mobility. The idea here is that you are still doing some form of exercise without stressing your body out too much, the same way that you would on regular training days.

Best Sleep and Recovery Habits

Track Your Sleep

Again, it's not just a matter of merely getting your eight hours every night. You should also be paying attention to the quality of your sleep. This is why it might be wise for you to invest in a sleep tracker. Most modern fitness tracking devices these days have a built-in heart rate sensor that can help track your sleep cycles at night. These devices will tell you how much time you're spending in each stage of a sleep cycle and how many cycles you go through every time you fall asleep. Tracking your sleep for the long-term will also give you a better picture of how your performance might be given certain sleeping patterns. Your data might tell you that you perform better during the day (and during training) when you get x amount of sleep a night.

Stay Away from Blue-Light Devices Late at Night

Unfortunately, we are surrounded by devices that emit blue light every single day. Your television screens, computer monitors, and smartphones all emit blue light. This blue light isn't just straining your eyes, they're also keeping you from falling asleep. This blue light sends certain signals to your brain that mimic the rays of the sun. So, your brain ends up getting tricked into thinking that it's still daytime even when you're supposed to be falling asleep already.

Don't Drink Coffee Beyond 2 PM

Caffeine is a stimulant that increases your heart rate and gives you energy. Having an increased heart rate and restless energy are two things that will keep you from falling asleep. Therefore, it should be common sense that you avoid taking any sort of caffeine too close to bedtime. The duration of the effects of caffeine can vary from person to person, but a general rule of thumb to follow is that you should never drink coffee beyond 2 pm, especially if you're looking to be in bed by nine or ten at night.

Avoid Taking Long Naps During the Day

Power naps are great so long as they are executed properly. When you are sleep deprived, it can really help to just take a few minutes during the middle of the day and have a good power nap. Power naps are micro sleeping sessions that will help recharge your brain in a limited amount of time. However, you should be very careful that you don't let these power naps last for too long. Remember our discussion about sleep cycles? If you get into the deep sleep stage, you will find yourself feeling groggy and disoriented when you wake up from your nap. This is why it's better for your power naps to never be longer than 30 minutes. Also, avoid taking multiple naps in a day. One should be enough.

Force Yourself to Wake Up Earlier

One of the major reasons people struggle sleeping at night is that they wake up very late in the morning. Then, since they wake up late, they have a lot of energy that carries over into the later hours at night - and the cycle goes on and on. You can break that cycle by forcing yourself to just wake up early one morning. Don't hit the snooze button. Wake up, get off your bed, and do something productive. Make breakfast. Go for a run. Take a bath. Do whatever it takes to wake yourself up. You will find it a lot easier to go to sleep early at night if you wake up earlier too. Again, avoid pressing that snooze button.

Sleep in a Cool Room

Science has shown that sleeping in a room with lower temperatures will lead to better quality sleep. You are less likely to be woken up in the middle of the night when you are in a cooler sleeping environment. Also, it's easier for your heart rate to get lower when you sleep in colder temperatures. This means that your body is more prepared to slip into the deep sleep stage of your sleep cycle.

Engage in Cross-Training

Do cross-training. Do something that your body isn't used to. It's important that you introduce new stimuli to your training regimen so that your body is constantly being challenged in new paradigms. Over time, even as you increase load and volume with resistance training, your body will reach a plateau. Go out for a run every once in a while. Join a yoga class. These are all great ways to really approach your fitness more holistically. It will also keep you from getting bored by doing the same routine over and over again.

Do a Proper Warm-Up and Cool Down During Every Training Session

Don't just jump straight into a lifting session cold. If the workout says that you need to do five sets of five reps of deadlifts at 225 lbs, then you need to make sure that your body is prepared to handle that workload. The first thing that you need to do is warm up by breaking a sweat. Do some dynamic stretches that will activate your muscles, finetune your range of motion, and increase your heart rate. After that, do some light reps of deadlift first and gradually work your way up to your first set at 225 lbs. This is so you don't completely shock your body into a stressful condition. It will also help ensure that your muscles are ready for whatever you're going to put them through. Then, after a training session, make sure to do a proper cool down. Do some mobility work by doing a few static stretches or by foam rolling.

Devote at Least 10 Minutes Every Day to Mobility Work

It just takes ten minutes every day for you to improve your mobility over time. We've already talked about how mobility can help improve your performance at the gym and can help prevent any unwanted injuries. Just take ten minutes out of each day to focus on a specific muscle group for your mobility. Prioritize areas that are closer to your major joints, such as your shoulders, hips, knees, and ankles. For example, today, you could work on your hip area. So, you should be foam rolling your quads, hamstrings, and glutes. That whole process will only require ten minutes. The next day, you can focus on your shoulder by massaging your pectorals, scapula, lats, and delts. Again, target different muscle groups consistently and your mobility will develop over time.

Reduce the Amount of Stress in Your Life

Lastly, just reduce the overall amount of stress in your life. Don't sweat the small stuff. If possible, try engaging in meditation throughout various points of the day. Remember to always keep things in perspective. Stress is known to have some very ill effects on your body's natural processes. You are already stressed enough at the gym when you go through hard workouts. That should be enough. Any other unnecessary stress in your life should be avoided at all costs.

Chapter 5

Training Your Muscles

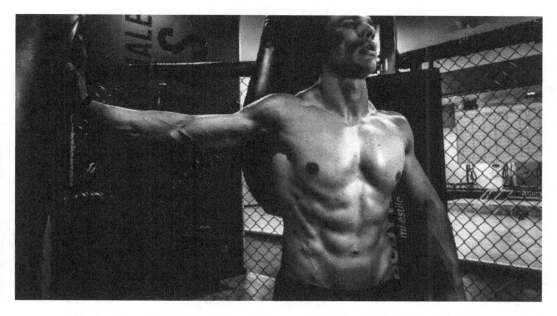

Now the time has come to talk about the exciting aspect of building your physique: training. There are some people who like to exercise and there are those who see it as a chore that they need to get over with. Regardless of how you view exercise in general, it's important that you have a very good relationship with whatever training regimen that you adopt for yourself. No two people should ever be given the exact same fitness and training regimen. There are a variety of variables that go into dictating what the perfect training pedagogy should be for you. However, it should be obvious that the more you enjoy and embrace your training, the more likely that you're going to be able to stick to it.

At the end of the day, that's the goal. You should be looking to build consistency with sustained efforts over a prolonged period if you want to see dramatic results. You can't expect significant progress in a short amount of time. This is why you need to adapt or build a training program that is designed for you to execute in the long term. Now, in order to do that, you need to orient yourself on the various movements that are involved in training your muscles. You have to start small. This chapter will help you learn all about the basic fundamentals of training specific muscle groups in order to stimulate growth and development. Once you have the knowledge on how to train specific muscle groups, you will also be taught about how you can string all of those different exercises together to create a cohesive and effective training program for yourself.

More than just learning how to make the most out of different exercises to stimulate muscle growth, it's also important that you know how to execute them properly. You must learn how to structure them into your program as well. If you perform a particular movement poorly, you could be doing significant and even irreparable damage to your muscles. If you're not structuring your program properly, then you might just be wasting all of the efforts that you're putting into the gym. It's imperative that you understand the nuances involved in structuring a strength training program so that you don't end up shooting yourself in the foot.

Before moving on, you should be proud of yourself for making it this far. Developing the resolve to pursue a greater body for yourself is something to celebrate. Unfortunately, not many are willing to put forth the time, effort, and commitment to pursue the best versions of themselves. By doing so, you are already separating yourself from the pack. You are a cut above the rest. Now, it's just important that you adopt the know-how that is necessary to get you to achieve your goals in the most efficient and effective ways possible. After all, none of this information is new or untested. This is knowledge that has been passed down by experts and enthusiasts over the years. Right now, muscle building is still a developing science and new breakthroughs and discoveries are being made every day. This is why it's important for you to continue to learn by reading books like these to help you stay safe and healthy as you train your body to its limits.

Compound vs Isolated Movements

Before we can get to the specific movements that are designed to stimulate muscle building, it's first important to identify the general classifications of these exercises. Generally, in any kind of exercise program, movements can be classified into one of two types: compound and isolated. Starting now, you should always be making it a point to prioritize compound movements as much as possible when adopting or creating a training plan. However, there should still be some room for isolated movements in your program as well. You will understand why as you learn more about the specific strengths and weaknesses of each movement category.

A compound movement is a type of exercise that requires the engagement or recruitment of multiple muscle groups found throughout various areas of the body. A classic example of such a movement is the deadlift. This requires the engagement of the core muscles, legs, and upper back. Another example of a compound movement is the pull-up which requires the engagement of the biceps, lats, and core. The reason that compound movements are much more beneficial for athletes is that they work multiple muscle groups in one go. This means that you're getting more bang for the buck with these movements. Also, compound movements tend to translate better into real-life strength. This means that they are more functional in nature and can help you get better with everyday tasks. For example, a deadlift can translate into helping you lift a big water jug or a piece of furniture off the floor. A pull-up can help you in situations where you might have to climb onto an elevated space using just your upper body. Aside from that, compound movements better develop your neurological fitness as well. Since you are working multiple muscle groups, your brain is getting its workout as well by trying to coordinate the proper function of these different muscle groups.

As you may have surmised, isolated movements are exercises that focus on single muscle groups at a time. They are designed to really target just one muscle group so that all of your attention is towards that specific area on your body. A classic example of an isolated movement is the bicep curl. A bicep curl, as its name implies, is a movement that only specifically targets the biceps. Obviously, the biggest disadvantage of an isolated movement is that you're not really getting the most bang for your buck. If you have a training plan that is composed purely of isolated movements, then it's going to take you much longer to complete a full body workout. However, that doesn't mean that isolated movements don't have a place in your training regimen. Isolated movements can be very effective for meeting specific goals such as correcting strength imbalances or weaknesses. This is a concept that is going to be discussed further in a later portion of this chapter.

Holistic Muscle Building

Now, it's time to talk about the importance of building your physique in a holistic manner. Too many times, people are guilty of avoiding working on their weaknesses and merely focusing on their strengths. This doesn't just happen in the realms of exercise and fitness. It happens way too often in various aspects of life. A writer who is skilled in writing romance will dare not practice writing fantasy novels. The martial artist who is good in boxing will be discouraged from engaging in wrestling drills. In bodybuilding, a person with strong legs is always going to prefer doing squats over pull-ups. As a result, they end up spending more time on the things that they are already good at just because they enjoy it more. This is the wrong approach to building your optimal physique.

An argument can be made that you should be spending more time on your weaknesses so that you have a more balanced approach to developing your body. If you know that you are leg-dominant, then devote more time and effort to working on your upper body. You don't want to end up having mammoth legs and toothpick arms, don't you? It's important that before you adopt a training plan, you assess your current fitness level first. Take a look at yourself in the mirror and perform an eye test. Does your body look proportional to you? Do your arms seem bigger than they should be? Is your waist a little pudgy? Are your legs smaller than the rest of your body? Once you determine what your strengths and weaknesses are, then you have a better idea of what you need to be working on when you make your training plan.

The Dangers of Muscle Imbalance

One thing that you must always be mindful of when you start your strength and resistance training is muscle imbalance. Too often, whether people are athletic or not, they go to visit therapists or chiropractors to help them with aches and pains in their body. A lot of the time, these aches and pains are brought about by muscle imbalances. Given that you're about to put your body through a stressful training regimen, you should expect that you would be more prone to developing muscle imbalances.

What is Muscle Imbalance?

To put it simply, a muscle imbalance is when one side of your joints exhibits considerably more strength than the opposing muscle on the other side of the joint. When talking in terms of physiology and biomechanics, this is not how your body should be structured or designed. When you have a muscle imbalance, this can be deemed as an abnormality that could potentially cause some serious complications in the way that you function biomechanically. When you have strength imbalances all over your body, one side could end up overcompensating for the other in order to cover that imbalance. This overcompensation could lead to potential injury and tissue damage.

What are the Symptoms of Muscle Imbalance?

Figuring out whether you have a muscle imbalance isn't always going to be so obvious, especially when you're doing it on your own. If you have a trainer who is watching you as you workout, they might have a better vantage point of spotting weaker areas in your body. However, if you're working out on your own, things might be a little more difficult as you have to engage in a high-level of self-assessment. Fortunately for you, there are ways in which you can test whether you have any existing muscle imbalances or not. Some of the most common symptoms of muscle imbalance include:

- lower back soreness/pain
- neck pain
- shoulder impingement
- knee pain
- rotator cuff tendonitis
- joint sprains
- tendonitis
- slipped discs
- muscle tears, etc.

Essentially, these kinds of injuries that seemingly pop out of the blue don't exist out of chance. They are there for a reason. You might be wondering what causes these little nagging aches and pains. Well, they could be caused by a number of possible reasons. But you should definitely be taking a look at any muscle imbalances that you might have

How Do You Address Muscle Imbalances?

Remember earlier when we talked about how compound movements are more efficient in helping you bulk up and get the body that you want? Well, that's still true. But we also talked about isolated movements and how they play a role in developing your overall strength as well. This is where they come in. The best way to correct muscle imbalances is to strengthen those weak muscles so that they are able to catch up to the rest of your body. Isolated movements that are designed to target specific muscles are great for correcting muscle imbalances. They are also great for providing accessory strength to your other compound movements which are inherently more complex.

For example, you might be doing a back squat and you notice that your legs are strong enough to push the weight up, but your core always gives in. You can then perform isolated movements that target specific muscles in your core to help you get better at a back squat. Another example of this is the pull-up. The pull up is a complex movement that recruits various muscle groups. There are some people who will find it difficult to perform a pull up properly because they are weaker in certain muscle areas. They might have enough strength in their lats to begin the ascent of a pull-up, but they might not have the bicep strength to finish it off. By doing bicep curls, an isolated movement, this can help correct the muscle imbalance so that the muscles recruited for a pull up will progress in a more unified manner.

Think of your muscles like a family. Every single muscle group is a member of that family and has some very specific roles to play when it comes to performing certain movements. When one member of the family is weak, then that compromises the performance of the entire family as a whole. Targeting your muscle imbalances is like finding the weakest link in your family and making sure that they aren't getting left behind. You always want to make sure that all of your muscle groups are progressing at a relatively proportional rate. As uncomfortable as it might be to confront your weaknesses, it's absolutely necessary that you address your muscle imbalances before they create any lasting negative impacts on your body.

Structuring Your Workout Plan

When it comes to structuring your workout plan, you have to keep in mind the various principles that we have discussed so far. To refresh, you need to prioritize compound movements so that your workouts and training sessions become more efficient. Next, you want to take a holistic approach to building muscle. This means that you never want to prioritize one muscle group over the other. Lastly, you want to avoid developing any muscle imbalances. This is why you need to create a workout plan that addresses all of your muscle groups and allows all of them the opportunity to grow and develop over time.

The first question that you might ask is how many times in a week should you be training. Well, the answer is going to be different from person to person. Again, it all depends on what your goals are and what your lifestyle is like. However, in general, you should shoot to have around four to five days a week of intense training if you're serious about building muscle. Again, it takes sheer will and consistency to achieve the body that you want. If it were easy, then everyone would be all chiseled up. Training sessions should typically be around an hour long. If you're efficient, you might be able to get things done in thirty minutes. It's all dependent on your level of fitness and how your body responds to training.

Push-Pull Movements

Aside from compound and isolation movements, we must also discuss push and pull movements. When talking about resistance training, your body is often doing either one or the other. It's either you're pushing against the force of gravity to lift a weight up or you're pulling against the force of gravity. A classic

573

illustration of this would be a push-up and a pull-up. As you start choosing the movements that will make up your workout plan, you want to make sure that you are adding healthy doses of both push and pull exercises.

You can choose to approach this in either one of two ways. One is that you can dedicate one training session to exclusively push or pull movements and then alternate these sessions over the course of the week. For example, Mondays and Wednesdays can be dedicated to pushing movements while Tuesdays and Thursdays can be dedicated to pulling movements. Then, Fridays can be dedicated to a combination of both. However, another approach to structuring a push-pull training program is by incorporating both movements into every training session. For example, you might plan to perform six different exercises for Monday. Three of those exercises would be push movements and the other three would be pull movements. Then, you would carry this kind of exercise format throughout the week.

You might still be wondering why a push-pull movement or workout scheme would be beneficial to you. Well, ultimately, the answer can be summarized to the following reasons:

Offers Optimal Recovery

We've already talked about how rest and recovery are very important aspects of building muscle. The push pull principle of training scheduling can help you structure your muscle recovery better. So, since you're splitting your training week into different segments (push and pull), then you're giving your muscles a chance to rest on days where they're not active. For example, if you are working on push movements on a Monday, then you are likely to engage muscle groups like quads, pecs, and deltoids. On

Tuesday, if you are focusing on pull movements, then you are giving Monday's muscles a rest because you're focusing on other muscle groups like hamstrings, biceps, and lats.

Promotes Muscle Balance

By properly dividing a training plan between push and pull movements, it lessens the chance of developing a muscle imbalance. When you follow the push-pull principle of training, you have to make sure that you are getting equal doses of every kind of movement. If you have three exercises that are devoted to push-centric muscles, then you should also balance it out by having three exercises devoted to pull-centric muscles. This way, it's a lot easier for you to find that balance whenever you're drawing up your training schemes.

Prevents Injuries

This particular benefit of the push-pull philosophy of training is merely a byproduct of the previous two listed items. First off, if you are giving your body a chance to have ample recovery in between hard training sessions, then you are lessening the chances of your body giving up as a result of overtraining. Also, we talked earlier about how having a muscle imbalance could lead to someone being more prone to injury. Since the push pull style of training lessens the chances of developing muscle imbalances, then it also negates any complications brought about by such a condition.

Provides Holistic Approach to Muscle Building

The push-pull method of training (paired with the integration of compound movements) can help you achieve a more holistic approach to muscle building. You would be able to target multiple muscle groups to make sure that every single area of the body is being given time and attention.

Saves Time

Lastly, it just makes your workout a lot more efficient. If you have a day job or a family, you don't want to be spending all of your time at the gym (unless you're a professional athlete). Ultimately, a push-pull philosophy can help simplify the way you structure your training so that you never have to rack your brain with thinking about what you're going to do on any given training day. So, aside from helping you be more efficient with your time spent at the gym, it also helps you be more efficient when you're plotting out your training schedule as well.

Upper Body Exercises

Your upper body includes all of the muscles that are found in your arms, upper back, chest, and shoulders. Functionally speaking, your arms are mostly responsible for lifting yourself up onto platforms or for moving heavy weight from point A to point B. There are a number of different upper body exercises that you can use for your training plan that are designed to target different muscle groups. Some of the most important compound exercises that you should integrate into your routine are going to be listed here.

Pull-Ups/Chin-Ups (Pull)

Pull-ups are a great pulling movement that helps build upper body strength. It's a movement that primarily targets your let muscles. But it also helps strengthen your biceps and forearms, depending on the positioning of your grip. If you grip the bar with your palms facing towards you, it recruits your biceps more than your lats.

Variations: Supinated Ring Rows, Lateral Pull Downs

Push-Ups (Push)

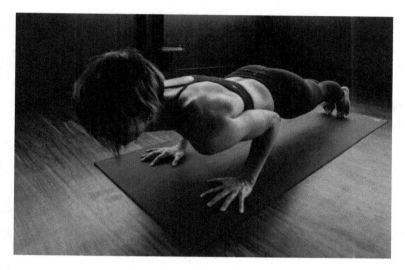

There are three major muscle groups that are being recruited to perform a proper push-up. For one, there are the pectoral or chest muscles. Then, there are the triceps, the muscles located at the back of your upper arm. Lastly, there is also the front of the shoulders or deltoids. The secondary muscle groups that are built by push-ups include the abdomen and the serratus anterior or wings. Like the pull-ups, you can change which muscles are being relied on depending on the positioning of your hands. A wider grip would place more emphasis on the chest while a closer grip places more emphasis on the triceps.

Variations: Push-Up on Ledge, Elevated Push-Up,

Handstand Push-Up, Knee Push-Up, Dips

Bench Press (Push)

The bench press functions the same way as a push-up and recruits the same primary muscle groups. However, it places less emphasis on the core as you don't have to be propping your body up. Also, like the push-up, a closer grip recruits the triceps while a wider grip recruits the chest. This movement can be performed with either dumbbells or barbells.

Variations: Inclined Bench Press

Shoulder Press/Military Press (Push)

A military or shoulder press is a movement that can also be performed with barbells, dumbbells, or even kettlebells. It mostly targets the deltoids or the shoulders and has a secondary emphasis on the triceps. By extension, especially if performed in a standing position, the movement will also recruit the core and legs for added stability.

Rows (Pull)

A row is a movement that is often performed with dumbbells or kettlebells. However, there are variations that also allow for the use of barbells. The muscle groups that are mainly recruited when performing a row are the latissimus dorsi, trapezius, and rhomboid muscles. There is also a secondary emphasis on the biceps and forearms, depending on the positioning of the grip.

Variations: Bent-over Barbell Rows, Plank Rows

Special Exercise: Thrusters (Push)

The last upper-body exercise listed here is special because it is technically a full-body movement. The thruster can be performed with either a dumbbell, kettlebell, or barbell. It involves combining both a weighted squat and a military press all in one swift movement.

Core Exercises

Sure, it would feel and look great to have a six pack. But that really isn't the best part about having a strong core. When one talks about training the core, not a lot of people necessarily understand what muscles are involved in core training. Most of the time, they might think of the upper and lower abs, and maybe even the side obliques. However, your body's core muscles also include your glutes and lower back. All of these muscle groups are in charge of protecting and stabilizing your spine. Without a strong core, your spine would be very vulnerable and this could lead to some very serious injuries, especially when you're lifting heavy weights. You should always look to incorporate these basic core exercises into your training regimen.

Planks

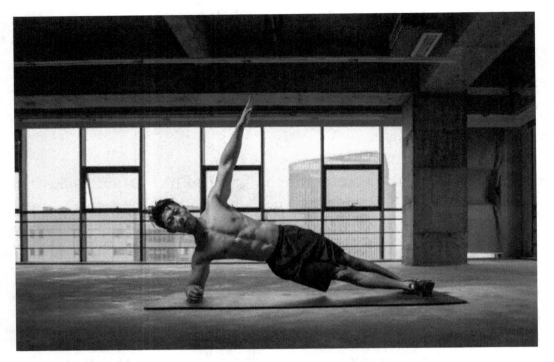

Many athletes and coaches will say that planks are the most efficient way to train your core. This is because the movement practically recruits every muscle group in your core region. It places a heavy emphasis on your frontal abdomen and your lower back. There is also a secondary emphasis on your gluteus maximus. There are also other variations of a plank that are more focused on the side obliques. Consequently, depending on how you position yourself in the plank, the movement can also improve shoulder stability.

Variations: Side Planks

L-Sits

The l-sit is one of the most complex core exercises because it requires a substantial amount of mobility and upper body strength to execute. Most people who are tight in the hips and hamstrings wouldn't be able to properly execute an l-sit due to their mobility issues. This is a movement that primarily relies on shoulder stability and pectoral strength for stabilization purposes. However, it requires a significant deal of abdominal and lower back strength paired with hip mobility in order to raise one's legs to a straight elevated position.

Variations: Hanging L-Sits, Seated L-Sits

Hanging Knee Raise

The hanging knee raise is a great core exercise that places a heavy emphasis on the frontal abdomen. However, it is also a great exercise for building grip strength and improving shoulder mobility. The general goal is to lift the legs by hinging at the hips and engaging the core.

Variations: Hanging Leg Raise, Toes to Bar

Back Extensions

Most core exercises tend to place a heavy emphasis on the frontal abdomen, side obliques, or the glutes. This is why it's important to incorporate back extensions into one's exercise routine as well because it targets the lower back, which is a part of the core muscle groups.

Sit-Ups

When you think of strengthening someone's abs, your mind might automatically picture someone doing a bunch of sit-ups. The primary muscle groups that are being recruited for a proper sit-up are the rectus abdominis, transverse abdominis, and obliques. Aside from that, sit-ups also help strengthen the lower back and hip flexors.

Variations: Crunches, Butterfly Sit-Ups, Weighted SitUps

Lower Body Exercises

People love showing off their biceps, back muscles, or abs whenever they've been working hard at the gym. Although, you might not realize that some of the biggest muscles in your body can be found in the lower body. Think about how much you use your legs on a daily basis. Whenever you jump, walk, stand, run, or do anything that involves you moving around from one place to the next, you are using your lower body. You wouldn't be as mobile as you are now without your lower extremities. This is why it's important that you pay more attention to training your lower body as well. It isn't just about having the biggest biceps in town. As they say colloquially, don't skip leg day.

Squats (Push)

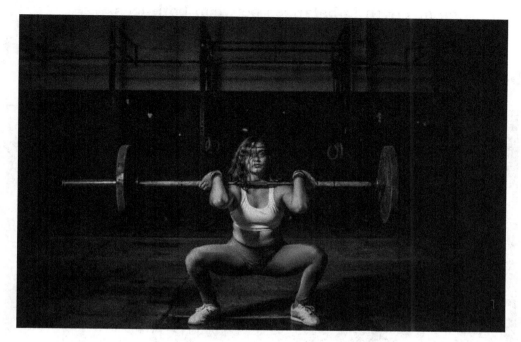

The squat is said to be one of the most important foundational movements that you could ever integrate into your workout routine. Having a strong squat translates to you having stronger legs that will serve as the foundation for whenever you stand, walk, jump, or run. The squat primarily recruits the quadriceps (front area of your leg), but it also has a secondary effect on your glutes, hamstrings, and calves as well.

Variations: Air Squat, Barbell Squat, Pistol Squat, Split Squat

Lunges (Push)

Lunges are like squats in terms of the muscle groups that they target. However, they offer a greater emphasis on single-leg engagement. This is an effective lower body exercise for addressing strength imbalances between both legs.

Variations: Walking Lunges, Reverse Lunges, Side Lunges

Deadlifts (Pull)

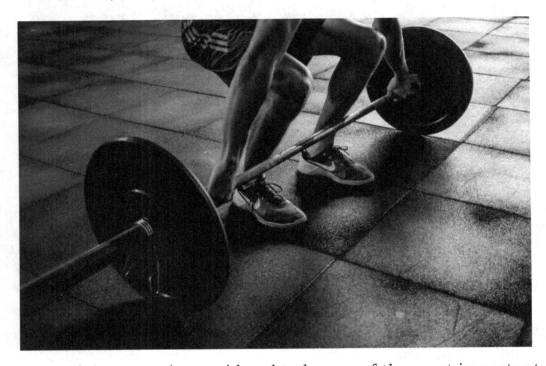

If the squat is considered to be one of the most important foundational movements in fitness, then so is the deadlift. Consider this as a pull variation of the squat, which is a push movement. The deadlift heavily targets the hamstrings, lower back, and glutes. However, it also requires substantial strength around the rest of the core muscles and the legs. Depending on how you position your feet, a deadlift can place heavier emphasis on a specific muscle group.

Variations: Stiff-legged Deadlift, Single-Leg Deadlift, Sumo Deadlift

Calf Raises (Push)

As its name implies, a calf raise is primarily focused on building up the calves. This is a very important exercise for those who are looking to build explosive strength that can translate into better running or jumping. Most leg exercises target the upper leg muscles like the quads and hamstrings. This is why it's important to integrate calf-dedicated exercises like the calf raise into one's bodybuilding routine.

Special Exercise: Cleans (Pull)

A clean is also technically a full-body exercise as it is a complex compound movement that recruits various muscle groups. The first phase of a clean is a deadlift that transitions into a powerful hip thrust paired with a violent shrug and pull from the arms into a strong front rack position. The first phase of a clean recruits the use of all the same muscle groups as a deadlift while the second phase of a clean recruits the same muscle groups as that of a row. The final phase or the catch position of a clean relies on pure core strength in order to stabilize the barbell.

Variations: Squat Clean, Power Clean, Muscle Clean, Dumbbell Clean

Special Note

Please remember that there are loads of different exercises and movements out there that can't be listed in this book for the purposes of practicality. Consider the movements listed here to be a list of capsule movements that you should have to serve as the foundation of your bodybuilding program. These are the foundational movements that will help you build that starting strength that you need to form good habits at the gym. Over time, as you become more

experienced in this field, you will be exposed to more complex variations and modalities. Always feel free to explore these new areas of fitness. Be bold enough to introduce new movements and rep schemes into your training regimen. This is all a part of the process of testing your body's abilities and seeing just how much you're capable of.

Incorporating Cardio

If you're an ectomorph, then try to limit cardio as much as possible. Don't spend more than thirty minutes a week doing cardio. That wouldn't be beneficial to your current fitness goals just yet. If you want to improve your cardiovascular health, then just opt for shorter rest times in between sets while lifting. This will cause you to have a more elevated heart rate while training and this can also serve as a good exercise for your heart while doing resistance workouts.

If you're a mesomorph, you will need to do more cardio than an ectomorph, but not so much. Spend around thirty minutes to an hour every week that's dedicated to pure cardio work. Whether it be a jog on the treadmill or a spin class. It's important that you keep your heart healthy and that you do some activities that will help burn away the fat. You have a thriving metabolism and you don't have to worry so much about getting fat unless it's likely that you might be in a constant caloric surplus. Cardio can help make sure that you don't go overboard with your calories so that you don't get any unwanted fat.

If you're an endomorph, as expected, you're going to have to do the most cardio out of all the body types. Since you're most likely to gain the most pounds, you might have to do a little more work at the gym to burn off some extra calories. You can do 30 minutes of cardio around three to four times a week just to be on the safe side. Again, it doesn't always have to be running on the road or on a treadmill. You can do spin classes, rowers, ellipticals, and other cardio machines. You can also opt to play cardio-heavy sports like basketball, tennis, or football.

Using Supersets

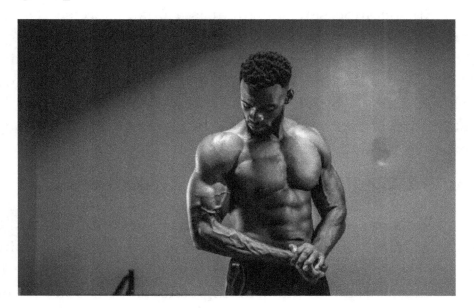

A superset is a common tactic that many lifters will use to introduce an added layer of difficulty and complexity to a workout. Aside from putting more stress on the body as a whole to produce better strength gains, it's also a more efficient way to go about a workout as it minimizes the amount of rest in between exercises. This way, athletes won't have to spend as much time as they need to at the gym.

The way that supersets work is that an athlete performs one set of a particular exercise and then quickly moves on to another set without any time for rest or recovery in between. The idea here is that it keeps the body constantly engaged and it trains the muscles to perform under stress. On top of that, it helps elevate the heart rate while performing resistance training exercises that usually don't have a cardiovascular component.

You can make use of the pull-push principle of training into your supersets by putting a push and pull movement against one another. For example, you might be using a squat as the first exercise in the superset. The squat is a push exercise. The next movement would be a row, which is a pull exercise. This is a great way to structure a superset because they offer different stimuli and both exercises recruit different muscle groups. So, while your lower body is recovering from the squats in the first set, you are still putting your body to work by using your upper body to perform the pull-ups.

Sample 1-Week Bodybuilding Program

Based on everything that you've been taught in this chapter so far, it's time for you to create or adopt a training scheme of your own. There are countless resources online that you can tap for ready-made training schemes. But it's also okay if you choose to make one on your own based on the knowledge that you have learned. It's also possible for you to find a ready-made program and tweak it a little bit so that it accommodates your own personal fitness level.

Here is a sample bodybuilding program that would be good for a week's worth of training. In this sample program, specific days are dedicated to push and pull movements with some days incorporating core training as well. You will also notice that during these exclusive push or pull days, there is a healthy balance between upper body and lower body exercises. Again, you want to make sure that you are taking a holistic approach to develop your fitness. It's important that you tackle different muscle groups. Also incorporated into this sample program are predetermined and mandatory recovery days. They are mandatory because that means that you have to rest on those days even though you might feel like you can go to the gym and lift. If you're feeling restless, then do some cross-training. Again, you shouldn't be training every single day. You need to give ample time for your body to recover in between long stretches of strength training. Feel free to take this sample program and adapt it to your own personal preferences.

Monday (Push + Core)

- Push-Ups - 3 sets of 12 reps
- Barbell Squats - 5 sets of 5 reps
- Military Press - 4 sets of 10 reps
- Calf Raises - 3 sets of 12 reps
- Planks - 3 sets of 1-minute holds
- Hanging Leg Raise - 3 sets of 15 reps

Tuesday (Pull)

- Chin-Ups - 5 sets of 7 reps
- Deadlifts - 5 sets of 5 reps
- Barbell Rows - 3 sets of 15 reps
- Cleans - 5 sets of 3 reps

Wednesday (Push)

- Bench Press - 5 sets of 5 reps
- Split Squats - 3 sets of 12 reps (each leg)
- Dips - 3 sets of 10 reps
- Lunges - 3 sets of 12 reps (each leg)
- Thrusters - 3 sets of 15 reps

Thursday (Active Recovery)

- Yoga, Swim, Run, Bike, or Mobility Drills

Friday (Pull + Core)

- Pull-Ups (or Lateral Pull Down) - 5 sets of 5 reps
- Dumbbell Rows - 3 sets of 12 reps
- Deadlifts - 5 sets of 5 reps
- Toes to Bar - 3 sets of 10 reps
- Planks - 3 sets of 1-minute holds
- Sit-Ups - 3 sets of 15 reps

Saturday (Active Recovery)

- Yoga, Swim, Run, Bike, or Mobility Drills

Sunday (Rest)

Chapter 6

Progressive Overload

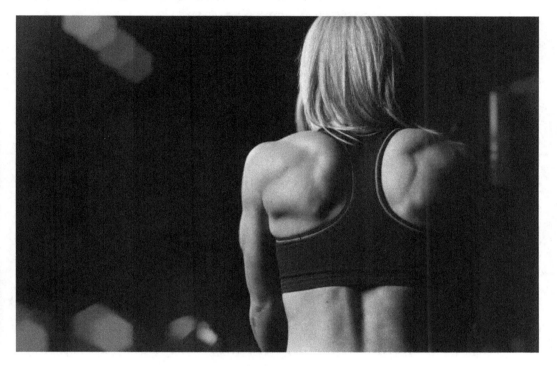

Let's say that you're done with finding a training program that works for you. You've done all of your research and analysis. You have already scoured the internet for many different workout programs and maybe you've consulted with licensed trainers or coaches to help you make a personalized program. That's great. But the job's not done. Learning and research do not stop. Just because you think you have a program that you're ready to start doesn't mean that you're going to be sticking to that program for the rest of your life. As you get better, fitter, and stronger, your workouts are going to feel a lot easier. When that happens, you know that it's time for a change.

One thing you have to know about the journey towards getting fit is that there is no destination. As cliche as it sounds, the journey is the destination. What this means is that the work is never really done. It doesn't matter how fit you become, there is always some work left to do. There is always going to be room for improvement. This is why you should be seeking progress, not perfection.

This chapter is going to help walk you through everything that you need to do AFTER you get started. Of course, getting started is a big step and you should always be proud of that. But it's not just about how you start. Results won't come just because you decide to get better with your fitness. Real results will only come if you continue to stick to the process and stay committed for the long haul.

What is Progressive Overload?

The whole principle of progressive overload centers around making your workouts more challenging over time. As you stay consistent with your training and workout regimen, your body is going to go through some amazing changes and transformations. You will find that things that you once found difficult are going to feel a lot easier and simpler to accomplish. However, while this might seem like good news, it's also going to be detrimental to your progress. The whole point of working out is challenging your muscles to the point of breakage so that there is ample space for growth and development. When there are fewer challenges, then there is also less room for growth.

Think of a first-grade student who is just being introduced to basic math. They learn about addition and subtraction. They might even learn about multiplication and division. As they learn about these concepts, they are making substantial strides from when they first started. Over time, with enough practice, they get better at developing their mathematical skills to the point where these concepts no longer prove to be challenging. When that happens, their growth stops. This is why second grade students will then be introduced to the world of fractions and percentages. This is to add another layer of complexity and challenge to the students and by extension, it also expands their room for growth.

It's the same as when you workout. Progressive overload isn't a principle that is only applicable to strength training or resistance training. If you're a runner, you practice progressive overload by increasing the speed or distance of your runs. This is a concept that can be applied to so many different disciplines. It's all because it's one that promotes perpetual growth and development by continually introducing newer and more challenging stimuli.

How Does it Benefit Your Training?

One thing that you should expect to experience whenever you engage in resistance training is a plateau. The success that you get from working out is going to deliver some very remarkable results. However, this success that you gain isn't always going to be linear in its rate of growth. In fact, there is a good chance that the fitter you get, then the smaller your gains will end up being. Ultimately, it might even get to a point where your body will begin to plateau. This means that you are no longer getting any gains or experiencing any progress whatsoever.

The main reason for this plateau can often be attributed to your rate of effort. Obviously, the fitter you get, then the less effort is required of you to complete certain physical tasks.

Pushing a 135-pound barbell overhead is going to be a lot more difficult at the start compared to when you're six or eight weeks into your training program. This is because you're getting fitter and the workouts are becoming easier. When your workouts get easier, you aren't really pushing your muscles to the point of breakage anymore. This is why progressive overload is the biggest tool that you can use to help combat whatever plateaus you might encounter on your road to fitness.

How Does Progressive Overload Work?

The concept of progressive overload is relatively simple. It's just a matter of you trying to find ways to make your workouts more challenging as you get fitter. Again, the fitter you get, the better you become at working out. This means that certain workouts that you did two or three weeks ago may no longer be as challenging now as when you first did them. So, you need to change these workouts up a bit in order to make sure that the stimulus still provides your body with a proper challenge. Now, how do you go about doing so? Well, there are three different approaches that you could take to introducing progressive overload into your training routine.

Increase Resistance

The first way to progressively overload yourself is to increase the level of resistance of your strength training. For example, let's say week one of the program had you deadlifting a barbell for five sets of five reps at 225 lbs. You repeat this cycle for maybe another week or two. Then, in the third or fourth week, you might find that these sets are a lot easier to accomplish and you're no longer challenged by it. You can make the exercise more challenging by increasing resistance or adding weight. In this case, you can up the weight to 235 lbs. This progressive overload is meant to adapt to your changing and improving level of fitness. Now, you might wonder about how much weight you should be adding. Well, it's going to be different for everyone as people tend to progress differently as well. However, a good rule of thumb to follow is that you should never look to increase the weight beyond 10% of what you were capable of lifting a week prior.

Increase Volume (Reps)

If you don't want to increase resistance, another way that you can go about introducing progressive overload is by increasing the volume of your workouts. If we stick to the same example of deadlifts at 225 lbs, you can still choose to keep the exercise at that weight as you get fitter. However, in order to progressively overload your system, you might want to increase the volume. So, try adding another set or a few extra reps for every set into your routine. Instead of five sets of five reps, maybe you can do six sets with the same rep scheme. You could also choose to stick to the same five sets, but with seven reps for each set now.

Increase the Rate of Work

Lastly, you could also opt to just increase your rate of work or productivity when you lift. Again, let's just stick to the same example of deadlifts at 225 lbs for the purposes of consistency. In the first week, it might have taken you around a full two or three minutes to recover in between each set. If you want to progressively overload yourself through increasing your rate of work, you can minimize the amount of rest that you take in between sets. By the fourth week, maybe your rest period in between sets would be around one minute to 90 seconds long instead of the two to three minutes you took when you first started. Even making this simple tweak can introduce a new stimulus to your body's muscular system and will offer the benefits of progressive overload.

Rules of Progressive Overload

By now, you should already have a good idea of what progressive overload is, why it's important, and how you're supposed to execute it. It's always good if you want to continue to introduce your body to new challenges, but you always have to be careful in doing so. By exposing your body to increasingly stressful environments, you have to make sure that you are keeping yourself safe and protected at all times. Progressive overload doesn't mean you going big whenever you're feeling confident. You still have to be methodical and tactical about it. Here are a few rules that you need to keep in mind when practicing progressive overload.

Always Start with Perfect Form

First of all, progressive overload should not even be an option for you if you're lifting with imperfect form. Again, if your form is bad, it doesn't matter how much weight you're lifting. You're doing it wrong and you're not going to get the gains that you want. Lifting with proper form means that you're engaging the proper muscle groups and that you're hitting all the right spots when it comes to your body's range of motion. If you can't perfect your form at lower weights or rep schemes, it wouldn't be wise for you to be progressing towards more challenging variations. There's no need to rush the process of progressive overload after all. Only move on when you're truly ready to do so.

Progressive Overload is Not a Linear Process

When you first start working out, you might think that you need to put the pressure on yourself to just keep on improving and improving at a rapid rate. In fact, you might create a schedule for yourself with regard to how much you should be lifting at a certain date. This is the wrong approach. You have to understand that your gains can't be scheduled. You shouldn't be giving yourself deadlines on how much weight you can lift. Progressive overload is something that you can only execute depending on what your body is capable of handling. It's not some kind of schedule that you NEED to adhere to in order for it to be effective. If your body is not capable of moving on from a particular level of resistance or volume, then stay at that level for a while.

Strength Gains Decrease Over Time and Increased Ability

Lastly, you have to expect that progressive overload is not going to become as rampant the older and more experienced you become in this field of fitness. When you're just starting out, it's very likely that you will experience significant jumps in your strength and abilities. This means that your progressive overload cycles might be a little more frequent. It's possible that you might be lifting significantly more weight in just a matter of one week. However, the more experienced and fitter you become, these strength gains become less and less frequent. There are some serious lifters out there who might even have to train a full year just to be able to gain 5 extra pounds on a single lift.

Chapter 7

Final Tips to Remember

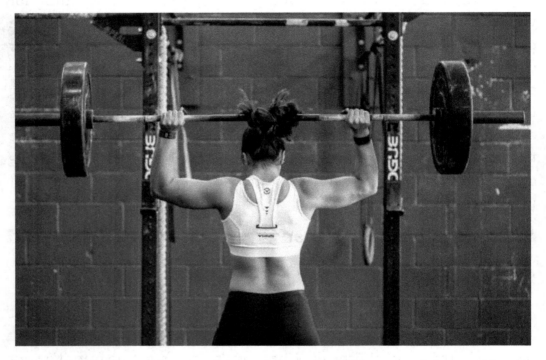

We're nearly reaching the end of the road here. You've come so far, but you still have far left to go. Fortunately, you know that you don't have to do everything on your own. Granted, this book might have been overwhelming to consume if you read it all at once. However, you will find that over time, with consistent practice, the knowledge in this book will become second nature to you. In fact, you might be able to write your own book on this topic one day. For now, just try to absorb little bits and pieces as much as you can and integrate these tidbits of knowledge into your daily training.

To conclude this book, here are a few key tips that you might want to keep to heart as you make your way through your fitness journey. Consider these tips to be the summary of everything that you've learned so far.

Don't Overtrain

Always make sure that you never overtrain. This means that you need to devote some time out of your training week to rest and recovery. Sure, you might think that doing more work will lead to more gains. That principle works only to a certain extent. Doing excessive work will not lead to gains. Rather, it will only lead to unwanted injuries that will sideline you and leave you worse off than when you started. Yes, you want to be giving it your best, but you don't want to overstretch yourself. In this case, it's better to work smarter than it is to work harder.

Leave Your Ego at the Door

One big mistake that amateur lifters or athletes make when they first start out is that they let their pride get to them. Sometimes, their pride will lead to them thinking that they're capable of lifting more weight than they can. What ends up happening? Injuries. Sometimes, their pride will have them believe that they are better or fitter than other people in the gym. This is the completely wrong mindset to have when approaching fitness. Your only goal at the gym every time you go there is to be better than the person that you were yesterday. Focus on that and the results will come.

Stay Consistent

Remember that old story about the tortoise and the hare? It's cool to be fast, but slow and steady wins the race. If you think that you can just go to the gym once or twice a week and give your maximum efforts for every session to get your desired results, then you would be mistaken. It would be a lot better for you to go to the gym multiple times a week and give small, but consistent efforts during every session. Eventually, these small efforts will add up to substantial gains that will only be given to you in the long run.

Don't Undereat

Even if you're an endomorph who is prone to gaining weight, it's important that you don't undereat. Of course, it should be obvious as to why an ectomorph shouldn't be undereating. Food is your friend, not your enemy. You need food in order to generate the fuel that is necessary for you to work hard at the gym. Without food, your muscles will not be able to grow and perform as efficiently as they should. It's all about moderation. You don't want to overeat, that's true, but it's just as important that you don't undereat.

Stay Hydrated

Always stay hydrated. Regardless if you're a serious athlete or not, you need water in order to survive. Whenever you put all of that hard work into your training, you are losing a lot of sweat in the process. You never want to end up feeling dehydrated as a result of your workout. Also, water is in charge of helping your body function properly, especially when it comes to processing nutrients from food. Water will help the protein synthesis process that is designed to help your muscle grow.

Prioritize Getting Quality Sleep

Sleep is a very undervalued resource that a lot of people take for granted. The amount of stress you put your body through as a bodybuilder is no joke. This is why you, more than most other people, need to devote more time to sleep. When you fall asleep at night, this is when your body is working double-time to revitalize and repair itself. Also, sleep is where you get a chance to regain your energy that will fuel you for another day of hard training.

Always Lift with Proper Form

Too many gym rats are guilty of this. Even people who have been working out for years can be guilty of this serious mistake. For the sake of completing a workout faster or for lifting heavier weight, some people will compromise their form in the process. This is a huge mistake because improper form while lifting (especially when the weights get heavy) can lead to serious life threatening injuries. You would never want to attempt a PR back squat without bracing your core. This would be the quickest way to damage your spine and potentially paralyze you. Exercise in itself isn't dangerous and it's not something that you should fear. You just have to make sure that you are keeping yourself safe and protected by lifting with proper form every single time.

Only do the Recommended Amount of Cardio

The topic of cardio is one that has been exhausted numerous times in this book. Again, there is no definite volume or amount of cardio that all people should be devoting to every day or week. It all depends on your physiological makeup and your personal goals. However, as a general rule of thumb, if you're looking to build muscle, you want to focus more on resistance training while limiting any aerobic activities like running. This is especially true if you are an ectomorph who has a tendency to struggle with gaining weight. Doing a substantial amount of cardio might prove to be counterproductive to your goals.

Stop Measuring Your Success Against the Success of Others

The thing you have to remember about your fitness journey is that it's yours and yours alone. Unless you're talking about your trainer, coach, or therapist, your personal health and wellness goals are not of other peoples' business. The same is also true for you. If you see someone at the gym who is not excelling as rapidly as you, don't make fun of them. They are on their own fitness journey and it doesn't concern you. It's also the same when you see someone who you think is doing better than you. Just because they might seem more successful doesn't mean that you should invalidate whatever success you have. Be happy with your successes and leave it at that. Stop comparing yourself to others.

Don't Be Afraid of Supplements

Lastly, don't be afraid of supplements. No, whey protein is not a steroid. No, creatine is not a performance-enhancing drug. Supplements are filled with essential nutrients, the same that you would find in the food that you eat every day. However, supplements should only be seen as supplementary products to your diet. Ultimately, your diet should revolve around whole food like meats, vegetables, fruits, and grains. You should only use supplements whenever you feel like you need a few extra nutrients that you find difficult to source from natural food.

Conclusion

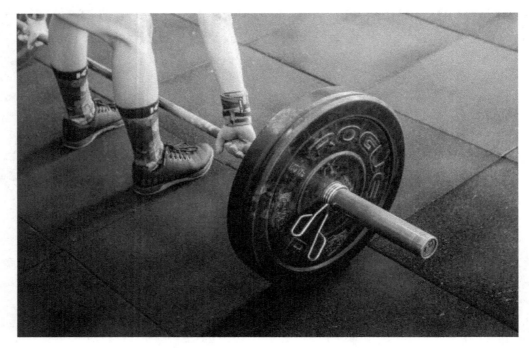

We're at the end now. Hopefully, this book will have inspired you to start strength training. At the very least, it should have added to your motivation to pursue a better version of yourself; the one that you deserve to be. Yes. You deserve to have the body that you want. Fitness is not a privilege or a luxury that is reserved only for those who are going to be blessed by it. Fitness is a right that you earn through sheer will, commitment, and hard work. Achieving fitness might not necessarily be easy, but it's always going to be possible. It doesn't matter what your background might be. Whether you had an athletic upbringing or not, you are still capable and worthy of pursuing and achieving your own personal fitness goals.

Too many people all over the world make the mistake of thinking that they don't have it in them to succeed. That's never the case. Improving one's fitness is a feat that is reachable and attainable for just about anyone. Even people with literal physical handicaps are capable of pursuing better versions of themselves. No, people don't lack the opportunities to become fitter. What they lack is the commitment and the willpower to actually pursue these goals.

You might have been guilty in the past of having a lot of excuses to not make the time for fitness. You were too busy. You felt like you didn't have the time. You didn't have enough money for a gym membership. These are excuses that all sorts of people have been using for the longest time now. Ultimately, what you have to realize about excuses is that you would never hear them from the people who genuinely want to make changes in their lives. This is because the people who are really willing to make these changes happen aren't going to be focusing on excuses. Rather, they focus on solutions. By reading this book, you are proving to yourself that you are shifting your focus towards the solution. You recognize that there is a problem and that there is room for improvement in your life. The fact that you're seeking out solutions is proof that you're ready to take that next big leap forward.

On your road to fitness, remember that you are going to encounter the occasional stumble. Success isn't going to come to you immediately and when it does, it isn't always going to be linear. You are going to have your fair share of ups and downs, just like in life. You might feel like you're taking two steps forward and one step back every so often. That's okay. That's perfectly normal. These kinds of slumps and setbacks are to be expected. They're not nearly as important as how you would respond to such occurrences whenever they take place.

Just remember that one of the most important traits that you need to develop here is persistence. There will always be a ton of excuses you can make for you to not get fit. There will be a variety of different factors out there that will discourage you from pursuing your dreams. You are bound to hit a few roadblocks that will just make you want to quit. But if you stay persistent enough, then none of these things will matter. They will merely be but a slight hiccup on your road to self-fulfillment.

As you go out and put forth the effort to get the body of your dreams, always stay confident in the fact that you are worthy of having such dreams, to begin with. Be proud of having the audacity to believe that you deserve to become a better version of yourself. This is not only beneficial to you, but also to the people who will see your work. You will serve as a light and inspiration to those who are afraid to start. Your spirit will become a source of empowerment and confidence for those who don't believe in themselves. That's also one of the best things about fitness. It's a community. Even though you might have your own individual goals and you mostly workout alone, you also know that there are other people out there who share similar struggles as you. There are also others who have dreams and goals that are just as big. Having that knowledge alone will give you a sense of solidarity from others in the fitness community to keep on going after what you want. And by actively participating in the community, you effectively do the same for the people around you as well.

I am CJD Fitness founder Baz Thompson, a CYQ Master Personal Trainer who has helped hundreds of people like you achieve their fitness goals. I work with professional athletes as well as coaching global executives and people of all ages. and I have enjoyed this opportunity to be working with you.

In closing, I would like to ask that if you have benefited from reading this book, and believe that others who have reached or surpassed age 40 and want to get into shape could benefit as well, please consider giving this book a favorable review on Amazon. This will send a signal to other potential readers who need help and will reassure them that this book is for them.

I trust you will experience excellent health and well-being on the long road of life that lies before you and wish you my very best. Thank you for letting me share my knowledge with you.

-   *Baz Thompson*

References

Aceto, C. (2020, January 2). 10 essential nutrition tips for beginners. Muscle & Fitness.

https://www.muscleandfitness.com/nutrition/gain-mass/top-10-beginner-nutrition-tips/

Behar, J. (2004, May 13). Rest and overtraining: What does this mean to bodybuilders? | bodybuilding.com. Bodybuilding.Com;

Bodybuilding.com.

https://www.bodybuilding.com/content/restand-overtraining-what-does-this-mean-tobodybuilders.html

Bubnis, D. (2020, July 30). Progressive Overload: What It Is, Examples, and Tips. Healthline.

https://www.healthline.com/health/progressiv e-overload

Butler, S. (n.d.). The Problem with Muscle Imbalances.

Www.Thejoint.Com. Retrieved October 16, 2020, from

https://www.thejoint.com/colorado/arvada/arvada-West-38021/188888-problem-with-muscleimbalances

Chertoff, J. (2019, February 26). Muscular hypertrophy and your workout. Healthline; Healthline Media.

https://www.healthline.com/health/muscularhypertrophy#how-to

Costello, J. (2017, October 12). 5 reasons why you should build muscle. ActiveSG.

https://www.myactivesg.com/read/2017/10/5-reasons-why-you-should-build-muscle

Creicos, B. (2014, September). What is your body type? Take our test! Bodybuilding.Com

Bodybuilding.com.
https://www.bodybuilding.com/fun/becker3.h tm

de las Morenas, D. (n.d.). Bodybuilding Sleep: How to Maximize Muscle Growth While You Snooze |

How to Beast. How to Beast. Retrieved October 16, 2020, from

https://www.howtobeast.com/bodybuildingsleep/

Ferruggia, J. (2013, November 14). How To Approach Cardio While Building Muscle. Muscle & Strength.

https://www.muscleandstrength.com/articles/cardio-building-muscle

Fetters, K. A. (2018, March 23). 11 benefits of strength training that have nothing to do with muscle size. US News & World Report; U.S. News & world Report.

https://health.usnews.com/wellness/fitness/articles/2018-03-23/11-benefits-of-strengthtraining-that-have-nothing-to-do-with-musclesize

Frothingham, S. (2018, November 12). What is basal metabolic rate? Healthline.

https://www.healthline.com/health/what-isbasal-metabolic-rate

Mason, A. (2018, May 15). Why simple push and pull workout routines are the best. Studio SWEAT OnDemand.

https://www.studiosweatondemand.com/ssodarticles/schedule-best-simple-push-pull-workoutroutineplan/#:~:text=The%20primary%20muscles%20in%20a

Mazzo, L. (2018, April 2). Why core strength is so important (it has nothing to do with sculpting a six-pack). Shape; Shape.

https://www.shape.com/fitness/tips/why-itsso-important-have-core-strength

T-Nation (2007, July 3). The push-pull workout. T-Nation.

https://www.t-nation.com/workouts/push-pull-workout

Nilsson, N. (2003, October 20). Weights Or Cardio: What's It Going To Be? Bodybuilding.Com.

https://www.bodybuilding.com/content/weights-or-cardio-whats-it-going-to-be.html

Quade, S. (2018, December 11). The importance of nutrition. Bodybuilding.Com;

Bodybuilding.com.

https://www.bodybuilding.com/fun/teenquade3.htm

Ring, S. (2017, March 16). The 10 do's and don'ts of mobility. Bodybuilding.Com.

https://www.bodybuilding.com/content/the-10-dos-and-donts-of-mobility.html

Tinsley, G. (2017, July 16). The 6 best supplements to gain muscle. Healthline; Healthline Media.

https://www.healthline.com/nutrition/supplements-for-muscle-gain

Trinh, E. (2018, September 21). Push-Pull Training 101: Everything You Need to Know. Aaptiv.

https://aaptiv.com/magazine/push-pulltraining

Van De Walle, G. (2018, November 19). Bodybuilding meal plan: What to eat, what to avoid.

Healthline.

https://www.healthline.com/nutrition/bodybuilding-meal-plan#benefits

The End

CPSIA information can be obtained
at www.ICGtesting.com
Printed in the USA
LVHW100840030621
689239LV00010B/767